# NURSE EXECUTIVE TOOLKIT
## FOR DISASTER RESPONSE

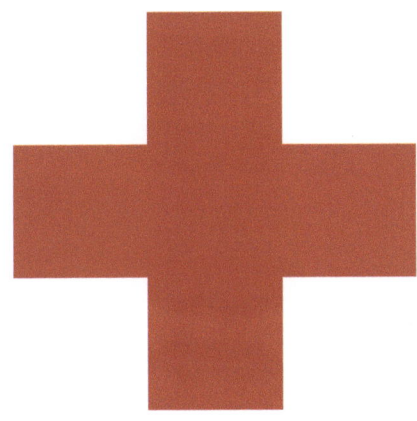

**DR. KATHY WAINSCOTT BERGER**
RN, NE-BC, BSN, MHA, DNP

JANUARY 2013

Copyright © 2013 Dr Kathy Wainscott Berger
All rights reserved.
ISBN-10: 1480277150
EAN-13: 9781480277151
Library of Congress Control Number: 2012921462
CreateSpace Independent Publishing Platform
North Charleston, South Carolina

# Table of Contents

Preface ................................................................................................................ v

List of Tables ..................................................................................................... vii

Introduction ....................................................................................................... ix

Chapter 1 ............................................................................................................ 1
The Role of Nursing in Disaster Preparedness and Response:
An Analysis of Practice and Competencies

Chapter 2 .......................................................................................................... 21
Program Plan with Needs Assessment

Chapter 3 .......................................................................................................... 45
Training Model

Chapter 4 .......................................................................................................... 53
Triage

Chapter 5 .......................................................................................................... 61
Capability Assessment

**Chapter 6** ........................................................................................................... 71
Program Evaluation

**Chapter 7** ........................................................................................................... 75
Quality of Care Degradation during Disasters

**Afterword** ......................................................................................................... 93

**Appendices: Resource Listing** ...................................................................... 95

    Appendix A : Federal & State Agencies/Organizations ................................ 97

    Appendix B: Academic Programs ................................................................. 113

# Preface

Recent disasters have created a whirlwind of change in the way health care is delivered during disaster response. Nurse Executives will be expected to direct nursing practice under conditions not encountered in normal daily operations. This book is intended to serve as a foundational resource for Nurse Executives to use in developing policy and program planning in order to more effectively deliver nursing care during a disaster. This book provides a list of competencies with measurement criteria, developed specifically for Nurse Executives, focusing on three domains of Administrative Leadership, Resource Management, and Professional Practice. This book also provides a capability checklist to use in assessing areas that need additional planning, divided into five categories: staff, space, supplies, communication, and patient movement. This book also includes a three-phase training plan and resource lists for agencies and organizations involved in disaster response on the national level, as well as individual states. The information and resources contained in this toolkit will support Nurse Executives in strengthening their abilities to deliver effective nursing care during disasters, when mass casualties and chaotic circumstances can easily overwhelm the health care system.

# List of Tables

| Table Number | Table Name | Page Number |
|---|---|---|
| 2-1 | Nurse Executive Competencies | 36 |
| 2-2 | Gantt Chart | 37 |
| 2-3 | SWOT Analysis | 38 |
| 2-4 | Sample Budget | 39 |
| 3-1 | Three Phase Training Model | 50 |
| 5-1 | Capability Assessment Checklist | 65 |
| 6-1 | Program SWOT Analysis | 73 |
| 6-2 | Program Evaluation Checklist | 74 |
| 7-11 | Ten Principles to Guide Resource Allocation | 88 |

# Introduction

The topic of Disaster Response has been ever present over the last few years and unfortunately we see the need for it on a fairly frequent basis. It is applicable to the health care community, just as it is to first responders such as fire and police personnel. In the past decade, beginning with the September 2001 terrorist attacks in the United States, our televisions, radios, and computers have broadcast photographs, reports, and live video of horrific scenes from disasters around the globe: collapsing towers in New York and the Pentagon in flames, hurricanes and flooding, earthquakes, tsunamis, tornadoes and additional man-made disasters such as train and plane crashes and gas attacks on subways. Once the initial shock of the event is over, the realization sets in that there are people trapped in those collapsing towers, people swept up in or stranded by flood waters, people crushed under heaps of rubble after the earthquake, people left to the elements when their homes were blown away by storms, and more people injured in train and plane wreckage. In fact, there may be so many people, with such numerous and serious injuries, that the medical community will be overrun with casualties. These people are first victims of a horrible event and, second, may be victims of a health care system that is not prepared or able to care for them.

Is our health care system prepared to handle disasters with mass casualties? If not, then what must we do in order to be prepared? How do we go about positioning the health care system and workers to be ready and capable for managing mass casualties? Who is responsible for leading these endeavors? What should the health care system and personnel expect during a disaster response? These are questions and themes found in the literature and on the minds of health care professionals across the globe. In this toolkit, these questions and themes are addressed, via chapters built around the framework of disaster preparedness and response.

As an initial step in investigating and studying disaster response, a gap analysis is critical, in order to gain a better understanding of what exists and what needs further attention. To address the question of where to expect leadership, Nurse Executives are identified as vital members, as they lead nursing practice. The Nurse Executive is a well-respected, principal member of the health care community and is in an ideal position to provide leadership and direction in such a weighty issue as disaster response. Since nurses are one of the largest contingents, if not the largest, of health care workers in the country, the Nurse Executive bears immense responsibility. Responding to a disaster and to care for mass casualties will require skill and aptitude not encountered in everyday practice. The health care system will be taxed and individual health care workers may be pushed far beyond their comfort zone, both physically and emotionally. There will be changes in practice and philosophy, changes in quality of care, and ethical situations that few health care workers have encountered before. Recognizing that many nurses, including Nurse Executives, may have little to no training in disaster response, a toolkit with a program plan and resources was felt to be essential for ensuring that the Nurse Executive possesses the competencies and skills needed

## Introduction

to lead nursing practice in such a strained environment as during disaster response.

The goal of this toolkit is to provide an evidence-based resource for the Nurse Executive, which includes a program plan and evaluation, training and triage models, capability assessment, and resource lists.

# Chapter 1

**The Role of Nursing in Disaster Preparedness and Response:
An Analysis of Practice and Competencies**

# Introduction

In recent years, disasters and emergencies have highlighted the need for well-prepared nurses. Much work has been done. However, there are gaps in knowledge and uncertainty as to what the roles, practice competencies, and preparation should be, in order to ensure that nurses are prepared. There has been work done by numerous groups, with varying foci, on nursing practice and roles in a disaster, as well as examination of, and suggestions for, competencies. There remain, however, many differing and disparate opinions on specific competencies, training, and just how to coordinate and integrate the role of nursing in disaster response. In this chapter, gaps, constraints, possibilities, and practice implications are discussed.

The morning of September 11, 2001 led to the identification of needed changes in the US, and medical readiness for this kind of extreme disaster was among them. In a few years, Hurricane Katrina would expose just how little progress had been made. Despite hard work from various disciplines, federal government interest and dollars, national media attention, and the best efforts of dedicated health care professionals and educators, there remains a lack of clarity and consistency with disaster preparedness and response. A few years later, some international disasters illustrated these same issues on a global scale. The earthquake and tsunami in Indonesia, the earthquake in Haiti, and most recently, the earthquake and tsunami in Japan and tornado in Missouri in 2011 clearly demonstrated the critical need for prepared medical personnel in a situation that easily overwhelms the medical system with mass casualties. Ten years after the 2001 terrorist attacks that energized the discussion for disaster response, there remains a concern that disaster response continues to lack standards. This has resulted in calls for international standards for more successful coordination of disaster responses.[22] The purpose of this chapter is to focus on nursing practice, in order to identify and examine gaps and challenges and to propose recommendations for the future.

## Early Works

Seminal work in this area was published by Gebbie and Qureshi[13] in a matter of months after the September 11 terrorist attacks and laid the foundation for developing nursing competencies. Within the year, other early works emerged, outlining preparations for disasters.[9,10] Not surprisingly, some of this work was produced by military nurses, who were more familiar with mass casualty situations. In 2004, additional competencies were developed, differing somewhat from the earlier ones. Both the quantity and content of the competencies had a significant range.[39] Public health nurses had earlier experience with examining practice and competencies due to disease outbreaks in communities, which were considered emergencies or disasters. Regionally, some nurses had exposure to disaster response, such as with Gulf Coast hurricanes.[28] This author spoke with several nurses and other medical personnel involved in the Gulf Coast hurricanes and subsequent response. Their anecdotal stories often recounted that the hospital facilities had disaster plans, but that they were seldom practiced, or practiced at such minor levels that it was all but a paperwork exercise. Also, the level of destruction was so severe and the time it took for help to arrive was so long, that it made the magnitude of the hurricanes and flooding overwhelming.

Additional work by Gebbie et al. addressed public health and individual competencies, including defining competency.[11,12] Others decided to actually put practice to the test and conducted some research. As part of developing a project for a community health nursing course, a private college in the southeastern United States held an actual mock disaster drill, encompassing countywide participation. This was one of the groundbreaking, multidisciplinary mock disaster drills of its kind. It highlighted the role of nursing in a disaster and the need for training to function under such circumstances. Emphasis was put on collaboration between various groups and agencies involved in the exercise. Subsequently, the post-drill evaluation cited it as the "most unified effort ever displayed in the community." It resulted in new partnerships that network to develop and support the community needs.[38]

# Recognizing Gaps

The gaps related to nursing practice and competencies range from inconsistencies in competency definition between organizations, to education needed, to basic terminology. The terms used in the milieu of disaster response include disaster, emergency, bioterrorism, mass casualty, and all-hazards response. However, there seems to be a lack of clarity as to the use of these terms.[29] Likewise, the establishment of competencies has significant variation. Weiner and colleagues at Vanderbilt University were involved early on with the development of the International Nursing Coalition for Mass Casualty Education (INCMCE), resulting in development of competencies and education modules. Although the INCMCE developed a rather detailed set of competencies in 2003, there are others which differ significantly in quantity and scope.[30] The INCMCE competencies are in line with the American Association of

Colleges of Nursing (AACN) practice for a general practice nurse, but other specialties are not included.[26]

Additionally, there is a lack of standards related to developing competencies.[32] Given that the profession of nursing strives to provide competency-based education, a lack of consistent and lucid competencies further complicates the issue for determining required education, training, and curriculum development. If education and training are developed and provided, how is its effectiveness determined?

Indeed, since the focus on emergency and disaster preparedness and response has largely occurred after the 2001 terrorist attacks in the US, there is a disparity in education and knowledge of those nurses trained prior to the more recently available information.[20] Numerous government and regulatory agencies, as well as professional organizations, including the American Nurses Association (ANA), have made recommendations for nurses to be trained in disaster preparedness, but this has proven to be a challenging task. The format, content, and availability of education and training changes frequently, due to revisions and updates, as well as to involvement from various agencies such as the Joint Commission, Department of Homeland Security, Centers for Disease Control (CDC), and the Federal Emergency Management Agency (FEMA).[30]

Despite the numerous recommendations for training and the multiple agencies involved, it is difficult to determine just how much progress has been made. The federal government has spent billions of dollars on training. However, there is no methodology or tool to assess metrics and outcomes.[29] There is a lack of evidence-based methods to deliver training or to verify whether training of health care workers actually improved their knowledge and practice skills. Emergency department staff who had received specific disaster preparedness training continued to voice uncertainty about their competence and abilities to function in such a situation.[4] A lack of assessment of those nurses who have been involved in disaster response has left a gap in potentially valuable knowledge and insight gained from such frontline experience.[28]

Finally, there are the questions of where responsibility for education should lie and who can provide it. When the Department of Homeland Security was created in 2003, jurisdiction issues came into play regarding training. The INCMCE task force survey of 455 nursing programs revealed concerns that 75 percent of the faculty was unprepared to teach this subject.[35] Even though there is widespread discussion and agreement that nurses should have training and be competent in practice during a disaster, how will it be accomplished when this large percentage of faculty are not prepared to teach this content?

## Constraints, Barriers, and Possibilities

Clearly, there are constraints and barriers with defining practice and establishing competencies. A myriad of questions exist regarding evidence-based education and practice: what competencies are relevant for varied nursing personnel and specialties; who should oversee or set mandates for education, training, and practice; and who will teach it? An additional confounding principle is a lack of research studies in disaster preparedness training. Much of the information available is informal work, which is not published and therefore not widely available to those entities making decisions and setting policy.[20]

As one author notes, nurses involved in a disaster are "pushed to extremes of scope of practice and beyond." The profession of nursing makes up the largest proportion of health care workers in this country and it is imperative that they be ready to respond and be able to provide care during a disaster.[15]

The potential for nurses to practice effectively during a disaster is enhanced through proper training and collaboration. Obviously, during a disaster, many other disciplines and agencies will be involved and nurses will be required to interact with them to manage patients effectively. Integration of efforts is enhanced when there is a multidisciplinary system in place. In fact, the ANA is one of eighteen organizations working on a national and regional framework for disaster response.[21] There are recommendations for nurses to participate in a minimum of one multidisciplinary exercise annually, in order to maintain minimal standards.[27] This could prove difficult for a variety of reasons. First, there are funding issues. It costs money to bring together multiple disciplines, with their equipment and personnel, in order to provide such an exercise. Second, staffing patterns and workflow in busy medical centers or clinics could be disrupted during such a drill. Finally, there is the issue of who would be responsible for organizing and establishing training content.

There are many players in this arena, all with their own agenda and focus. To illustrate the complexity: there are multiple specialties in nursing; regulatory bodies; local, state, and federal governmental agencies; professional organizations; academic organizations; and individual health care facilities, all of whom have varying responsibilities and foci on how to establish practice that fits their mission. Each has a very important piece of this complicated issue. The key is to defragment and reassemble the multiple pieces into a workable, evidence-based model. It's an odd paradox of having numerous agencies and organizations involved and making recommendations, while really none is clearly the pilot at the controls.

Further possibilities exist in learning from the international community, where nurses have had experience with disasters, such as in Israel, Japan, and Ireland. Interestingly, Ireland was the first location for a disaster nurse program.[34] Recent world events that have been on the news daily include natural disasters in several locations in Asia, plus war zones and terrorist attacks. The nurses in those locations would surely have rich and detailed experience and lessons learned to share with fellow nurses globally.

## Real World Disasters and Lessons Learned

To illustrate the challenges, scope, and magnitude of chaos and overwhelmed systems capabilities, some recent disasters will be reviewed. In 2004, a 9.0 magnitude earthquake and tsunami struck Indonesia, which killed over 100,000 people and left hundreds of thousands more injured and homeless. Lessons learned from this disaster had a recurring theme of response capabilities. Gaps in joint work and coordination between groups hampered efforts. Areas for improvement were identification of local experts who had knowledge of international standards and coordination of efforts within government agencies and the international community, which would enhance response. Water, sanitation, diseases, and mental health issues were identified as major problem areas in this disaster, as well as inequities in resources between urban and rural areas.[19]

In January 2010, a devastating earthquake of 7.0 magnitude struck Haiti, leaving parts of that country in near total destruction, including medical capabilities. The US Navy deployed its hospital ship, the *Comfort*. The summary from medical staff aboard ship included having patients arrive with no medical records or history. Many arrived in serious condition and in such a volume that made a comprehensive exam impractical. Other challenges included serious infections, wound infestations with worms and maggots, tetanus, and multidrug-resistant bacteria. Crush injuries were prevalent, which led to renal failure, which quickly stressed their dialysis capability with the supplies on hand. Overall, the volume of serious trauma, including multiple fractures, overwhelmed medical capabilities in what the staff termed a "flood" of casualties.[2] Another international team was deployed, the Israel Defense Forces Medical Corps Field Hospital, which came prepared to provide numerous levels and types of care. Because of their level of training and readiness, they were able to arrive in Haiti and have a field hospital set up within eighty-nine hours of the earthquake. This group was quickly saturated with casualties as well and was at full capacity within two days, seeing large numbers of trauma, infections, and surgical cases. Due to the limited resources, which were outstripped by the enormous numbers of casualties, limits had to be set on which and how many patients they could treat.[17] This brought to the fore the challenge of ethical considerations when demand outpaces supply. The Israeli group had to re-set priorities and implement a triage system that would determine not the level of treatment, but rather if the patient would be treated and who would be denied treatment. Although this is contrary to what most medical professionals are accustomed to or comfortable with, it was necessary to optimize the resources available.[23] These two groups of medical professionals were well trained and prepared for such situations, and yet even they were overwhelmed. It is important to note that field or pre-hospital triage is not the typical triage seen in hospital emergency rooms. Field triage using a START model identifies patients in one of four categories: deceased, immediate, delayed, or minor.

The next disaster was the earthquake with subsequent tsunami in Japan, March 2011. This island nation is used to earthquakes and prepares for tsunamis, but this one was of such magnitude that the damage was well beyond what was anticipated. The following accounts give a glimpse into just what the casualties and those medical staff attempting to treat them had to endure. In one town the hospital recounted that within a half hour they had near total losses of their food and medicine, because those items were stored on the ground floor and it was flooded by the tsunami waves. They had no power, running water, or heat. The temperature was near freezing, the bathrooms were overwhelmed, and there was no government assistance for a few days. Medical equipment had been damaged and part of the hospital had collapsed. The nurses were trying to clean muddy packages of medications and intravenous fluids by using alcohol. All they had to eat was some frozen vegetables. At the government-run elderly center, food was also running low and the daily allotment was two rice balls.[24] Another group recounts that they had no electricity, gas, or running water for two weeks. Several patients died because of the freezing temperatures at night. Bed linens and clean laundry were in short supply. Once they acquired a generator, they had two hours of power every evening, during which time the doctors tried to perform essential tasks. They also made use of a garden solar light to make rounds. Gasoline was in short supply nationwide, so transportation was problematic. Many of the nurses were working eighteen-hour shifts.[18] Lessons learned here included closer attention to where and how supplies are stored and how to prepare for operations during inclement weather without power or readily available assistance from governmental agencies.

Closer to home, a massive tornado struck Missouri in 2011, which all but leveled the town of Joplin. The hospital was so heavily damaged that it had to be evacuated. The windows were blown out, walls knocked down, some parts of the hospital caught fire, and x-rays and medical records got sucked up in the tornado and were found several counties away. This was a 367-bed hospital, which the staff was able to evacuate in ninety minutes, moving patients by whatever means possible, including sliding mattresses down stairs since the elevators were not functional. A triage center was set up in the parking lot, despite damaged cars, their smashed helicopter, and scattered debris.[6] Tragically, five patients in the hospital died, who were on ventilators. They lost power when the generator was sucked out of the hospital and there was no power source for the ventilators or oxygen.[25] Lessons from this experience included the need for alternate power sources and, on the positive side, the ability to evacuate a damaged hospital rapidly and to set up contingency operations.

A common thread in the literature regarding disaster preparedness and response is that many communities and areas depend on outside agencies or the federal government. This usually does not happen immediately and communities should plan to provide immediate care until external help arrives, usually in three to five days. Increased training for personnel and collaborated efforts, information, and communication management are essential for effective response.[16,31] Lack of integrated efforts and lack of international medical standards for care during a disaster response were cited as areas for improvement in worldwide disasters. Effective and timely information sharing and connectivity were also identified as needing improvement.[3,22] Interestingly, new communication methods have come into existence and are being used in disaster responses. During wildfires in California in 2007, the social networking service Twitter was used to communicate and update officials on fire locations and rescue center capacity. Blogs on Twitter provided real-time communication and enhanced collaboration and communication between firefighters, responders, local radio stations, and the public.[33]

## Practice Implications

Implications can be divided into three categories: definition of practice/competency, preparation/regulation, and policy. It is clear that nursing practice during a disaster or emergency will differ greatly from general day-to-day practice in the usual setting. Role definition is crucial. Understanding roles within a collaborative network, teamwork with other health care providers, and practice objectives are vital to successful outcomes during a disaster or emergency situation.[1,8,36,37] Developing a national certification, with establishment of competencies, would be a major step toward a more cohesive standard of practice. Certification would lend credibility to the importance of recognizing the uniqueness of disaster response nursing practice.

Preparation for disasters in the form of education and training is a critical element. There have been some proposals for regulatory bodies, such as state boards of nursing, to stipulate education requirements.[26] One example of this would be requiring this content in baccalaureate programs and requiring a specific number of continuing education credits per licensing cycle. Other proposals include the development of competency-based education, which can be established at local, regional, national, or international levels.[7,35] Additional regulatory possibilities are guidelines from the state level on the nurse's responsibility for volunteer registration and responsibilities during a disaster.[15] Research development is needed in order to evaluate and validate preparation and education.[29] Further research is vital in order to make progress toward sound, evidence-based decisions in this area. Since the focus on the nursing role during disasters is fairly recent, research studies are lacking in the literature. Additional guidance could be derived through position papers developed by professional organizations that provide more definitive guidance on education and in developing standardized curriculum content for basic nursing programs.

Finally, it is important to be aware of the political and policy components related to disaster response. Therefore, it is imperative that nurse leaders be involved in policy planning.[5,14] Financial and funding issues fall within the political and policy arena and we cannot forget this business perspective. Nurse leaders should be involved at the local, state, and national levels for policy development. Political decisions regarding research, grants, and educational funding need to have a nursing voice present as part of the discussion. Regulatory decisions about licensure and credentialing requirements, certifications, and continuing education are important components that will affect nursing practice. Nursing needs to be at the table of policy-making at all levels, concerning practice, academic, and regulatory issues.

## Summary

The importance of defining practice and establishing competencies cannot be overstated. These are crucial to the successful management of a disaster. We need to be effective partners in the health care community during disaster and emergency response. Nurses need to be educated, to know their roles, and to be able to function competently in that capacity. Otherwise they will be ill-prepared to deliver care to the masses of casualties who need nursing expertise and skills during a time of chaos.

# References

1. Akins, R., Williams, J., Silenas, R., & Edwards, J. (2005). The role of public health nurses in bioterrorism preparedness. *Disaster Management and Response, 3*, 98-105.

2. Amundson, D., Dadekian, G., Etienne, M., Gleeson, T., Hicks, T., Killian, D., ... Miller, E. (2010). Practicing internal medicine onboard the USNS COMFORT in the aftermath of the Haitian earthquake. *Annals of Internal Medicine, 152*, 733-737.

3. Baker, D. & Refsgaard, K. (2007). Institutional development and scale matching in disaster response management. *Ecological Economics, 63*, 331-343.

4. Becker, S. & Middleton, S. (2008). Improving hospital preparedness for radiological terrorism: Perspectives from emergency department physicians and nurses. *Disaster Medicine and Public Health, 2*, 174-184.

5. Chan, J. (2008). Politics and disaster response: Recent experience in Asia. *Disaster Medicine and Public Health Preparedness, 2*, 136-135.

6. Chaos, bravery in storm-struck Joplin hospital. Retrieved June 16, 2011 from: http://www.cbsnews.com/stories/2011/05/24/earlyshow/main20065622.shtml.

7. Coule, P., Schwartz, R. & Swienton, R. (2008). Emergency medical consequence planning and management for national special security events after September 11: Boston 2004. *Disaster Medicine and Public Health Preparedness, 2*, 134-135.

8. Danna, D., Bernard, M., Jones, J. & Matthews, P. (2009). Improvements in disaster planning and directions for nursing management. *Journal of Nursing Administration, 39*, 423-431.

9. Drenkard, K., Rigotti, G., Hanfling, D., Falhgren, T. & LaFrancois, G. (2002). Healthcare system disaster preparedness, Part 1: Readiness planning. *Journal of Nursing Administration, 32,* 461-469.

10. Fahlgren, T., Drenkard, K. & Neil K. (2002). Healthcare disaster preparedness, Part 2: Nursing executive role in leadership. *Journal of Nursing Adminstration, 32,* 531-537.

11. Gebbie, K. & Merril, J. (2002). Public health worker competencies for emergency response. *Journal of Public Health Managed Practice, 8,* 73-81.

12. Gebbie, K., Merrill, J., Hwang, I., Gupta, M., Btoush. R. & Wagner, M. (2002). Identifying individual competency in emerging areas of practice: An applied approach. *Qualitative Health Research, 12,* 990-999.

13. Gebbie, K. & Qureshi K.(2002). Emergency and disaster preparedness. *American Journal of Nursing, 102,* 46-51.

14. Gebbie, K. & Qureshi, K. (2006). A historical challenge: Nurses and emergencies. *The Online Journal of Issues in Nursing, 11,* 2.

15. Hale, J. (2008). Managing a disaster scene and multiple casualties before help arrives. *Critical Care Nursing Clinics of North America, 20,* 91-102.

16. Harrald, J. (2009). Review of disaster response and homeland security: What works, what doesn't. *Journal of Homeland Security and Emergency Management, 6,* 11, 1-3.

17. Kreiss, Y., Merin, O., Peleg, K., Levy, G., Vinker, S., Sagi, R., ... Ash, N. (2010). Early disaster response in Haiti: The Israel field hospital experience. *Annals of Internal Medicine, 153,* 45-48.

18. Japan: Deadly cold weather strikes tsunami-hit hospital. Retrieved June 16, 2011 from: http://reliefweb.int/node/392967.

19. Leitmann, J. (1007). Cities and calamities: Learning from post-disaster response in Indonesia. *Journal of Urban Health; Bulletin of the New York Academy of Medicine, 84,* 144-153.

20. Littleton-Kearney, M. & Slepski, L. ( 2008). Directions for disaster nursing education in the United States. *Critical Care Nursing Clinics of North America, 20,* 103-109.

21. Lyznicke, J., Subbarao, I., Benjamin, G. & James, J. (2007).Developing a consensus framework for an effective and efficient disaster response health system: A national call to action. *Disaster Medicine and Public Health Preparedness, 1,* S51-S54.

22. McCann, D. & Cordi, H. (2011). Developing international standards for disaster preparedness and response: How do we get there. *World Medical & Health Policy,* 3, 5.

23. Merin, O., Ash, N., Levy, G., Schwaber, M. , & Kreiss, Y. (2010). The Israeli field hospital in Haiti: Ethical dilemmas in early disaster response. *New England Journal of Medicine, 362,* e38.

24. Misery at Japan's tsunami-ravaged hospitals (2011). Retrieved June 16, 2011 from: http://www.cbsnews.com/stories/2011/03/14/501364/main20042841.html.

25. Murphy, K. (2011). Five patients who died in Joplin hospital suffocated. Retrieved June 16, 2011 from: http://www.reuters.com/article/2011/05/24/us-usa-weather-tornadoes-hospital-idUSTRE74N.

26. Polivka, B., Stanley, S., Gordon, D., Taulbee, K., Kieffer, G., & McCorckle, S. (2008). Public health nursing competencies for public health surge events. *Public Health Nursing, 25,* 159-165.

27. Rebmann, T. (2006). Defining bioterrorism preparedness for nurses: Concept analysis. *Journal of Advanced Nursing, 54,* 623-632.

28. Rebmann, T., Carrico, R. & English, J. (2008). Lessons public health professionals learned from past disasters. *Public Health Nursing, 25,* 344-352.

29. Slepski, L. (2005). Emergency preparedness: Concept development for nursing practice. *Nursing Clinics of North America, 4,* 419-430.

30. Smith, R. (2007). Making a case for integration of disaster-preparedness content in associate degree programs. *Teaching and Learning in Nursing, 2,* 100-104.

31. Smith, S., Gorski, J. & Vennelakanti, H. (2010). Disaster preparedness and response: A challenge for hospitals in earthquake-prone countries. *International Journal of Emergency Management, 7,* 209-220.

32. Stanley, J. (2005). Disaster competency development and integration in nursing education. *Nursing Clinics of North America, 40,* 453-467.

33. Veinott, B., Cox, D., & Mueller, S. (2009). Social media supporting disaster response; Evaluation of a lightweight collaborative tool. *The British Computer Society, 9,* 307-308.

34. Weiner, E. (2005). A national curriculum for nurses in emergency preparedness and response. *Nursing Clinics of North America, 40,* 469-479.

35. Weiner, E. (2006). Preparing nurses internationally for emergency planning and response. *The Online Journal of Issues in Nursing, 11*, 4.

36. Wetta-Hall, R., Fredrickson, D., Ablah, E., Cook, D., & Molgaard, C. (2006). Knowing who your partners are: Terrorism-preparedness training for nurses. *The Journal of Continuing Education in Nursing, 37*, 106-112.

37. Williams, J., Nocera, M., & Casteel, C. (2008). The effectiveness of disaster training for health care workers: A systematic review. *Annals of Emergency Medicine, 52*, 211-222.

38. Wise, G. (2007). Preparing for disaster: A way of developing community relationships. *Disaster Management and Response, 5,* 14-17.

39. Wisniewski, R., Dennik-Champion, G. & Peltier, J. (2004) Emergency preparedness competencies, assessing nurses' educational needs. *Journal of Nursing Administration, 34*, 475-480.

# Chapter 2

**Program Plan with Needs Assessment**

# Introduction

This program utilizes the Nurse Executive Toolkit for Disaster Response. Within this program, the Nurse Executive will address competencies that are necessary to deliver effective and efficient nursing care during a disaster situation. Disaster response is a recently identified focus for integration into nursing practice and in order to do so, competencies need to be developed. Contained in this chapter are theoretical models that have been identified to advance this program. Included are program planning, evidence-based practice, and change models, which provide a strategic, systematic approach. A needs assessment and supporting literature are included, as well as a SWOT analysis and a budget. Defining attributes of this program are effective planning and evaluation, successful implementation of evidence-based practice ingrained in competencies, and a genre of change that will spread innovation over time and be successfully adopted.

# NEEDS ASSESSMENT

## Executive Summary

Competency is defined in the dictionary as having suitable skill, proficiency, or expertise for a certain purpose, especially measured against a standard.[7,26] Establishing competencies is therefore an integral part of defining nursing practice. Measurement against a standard is especially important in a scientific field such as nursing, and is apropos to evidence-based practice. It is imperative that Nurse Executives have the tools necessary for competent practice related to disaster preparedness and response. As this is a fairly recent focus in the healthcare professions and not historically taught as part of standard curriculum in the academic setting, it is up to those Nurse Executives in leadership roles to be prepared to function in such chaotic and unusual circumstances. This program will provide the Nurse Executive with the necessary tools and planned strategies in order to accomplish this crucial undertaking.

## Mission

The mission of this program is to provide nursing leadership in the acute care hospital with the necessary tools to address competencies for nursing practice related to disaster preparedness and response. The Nurse Executive Toolkit for Disaster Response will serve the nursing leaders, but ultimately the patients who receive care during a disaster situation. The goal of the program is to provide a toolkit of resources and a program plan to enable the Nurse Executive to plan and manage nursing care effectively during a disaster.

## Vision

A standardized and evidence-based approach for nurse leader competencies will be provided via a toolkit for the Nurse Executive. This will result in greater proficiency in managing nursing practice during a disaster situation.

## Assessment of Needs

Four types of needs were assessed to understand the need for nursing practice definition and establishing competencies for disaster preparedness and response. Normative need is supported and defined in current literature. There is a recognized need for defining nursing practice and competencies for disaster response. It is also recognized that competencies discussed in the literature are often widely varied in nature, scope, and complexity and are frequently geared toward the agency or organization mission and goals and not specifically to the discipline of nursing.[8,9,11,25] The expressed need can be observed by the target audience, in that there is behavioral display of seeking resources to develop and define nursing competencies. A relative need identifies a gap between groups. This can be demonstrated by comparing acute care nursing and the lack of clearly defined competencies in that practice, with that of public health nursing, which defined their early on role and established competencies related to disasters and emergencies.[1,18,20] Finally, there is a perceived need. A survey questionnaire was developed and sent to a focused group of ten nursing leaders at hospitals in six states; eight of those completed the survey. This survey clearly showed that there is a perceived need for nursing to establish competencies. Results of the survey revealed that disaster response resources were not readily available, although the need to have such resources and role definition was important.

## Application

The needs assessment was conducted using an Asset Model approach. The focus of this model is to consider the assets, resources, and abilities that are already in existence and available.[12] The key then will be how to mobilize, organize, and put the existing capital into action. This model is applicable to establishing competencies for disaster response in that the available resources of nursing leaders and some general knowledge of disasters already exist. It is now a matter of bringing these resources together to implement defined competencies.

## Analysis/Conclusion

The needs assessment gives a clear picture of the necessity of disaster response nursing competencies. Within the constructs of nursing practice, having established competencies will further define nurse leader practice and develop Nurse Executives who are better prepared and more capable in managing disaster situations. The need to be prepared and to be able to function during a chaotic situation is paramount to delivering effective care.[6,15,16] The time to determine what competencies are needed is not during a disaster, but long before.[21,25,30] By applying the Asset Model and mobilizing current assets, nursing practice can be strengthened. A toolkit for Nurse Executives will provide an organized, evidence-based resource, which nursing leaders can use to maximize their nursing practice.

# PROGRAM PLAN

## Relevant Models and Theories

*Program Planning Model*

Issel[12] presents a framework for program planning. Program theory contains three components: the process theory, the effect theory, and their outputs. The logic model of program theory gives a schematic depiction of the subcomponents of each of the main two components. First, under process theory, the organizational plan considers personnel, resources, and infrastructure. Under effect theory, the service utilization plan considers the logistics of delivery, including marketing the program and examination of the program availability and accessibility. The literature supports using a clearly defined, logic model to plan and evaluate programs. One of the primary benefits is the identification of key stakeholders and a clear articulation of a common understanding of and vision for the program.[10] Identifying goals and objectives and then mapping a pathway, including resources and infrastructure, will lead to a more cohesive process and stakeholder buy-in.[24] A key point made in the program theory plan is that both of these components can evolve and change and may need adjustments during the planning phase. This plan is applicable to the program plan for a Nurse Executive toolkit for disaster response competencies because it addresses the organizational element and the service utilization piece necessary for final output or product. The Nurse Executive will need to identify and consider what infrastructure and resources are required to develop and build a plan for nursing, as well as what interventions are needed to deliver that plan.

## Evidence-Based Practice Model

Kitson's model, as listed in Melynk and Fineout-Overholt,[17] is a multidimensional model. This model, known as the Promoting Action on Research Implementation in Health Services (PARiHS) framework, is depicted by the following formula: SI=f (E, C, F). In this formula, SI=successful implementation, f=function of, E=evidence, C=context and F=facilitation. This model has an emphasis on organization and context is of central importance. It explains that practice is a function (f) of the nature of the evidence (E), the context (C) in which change will be introduced, and the facilitation (F) used to implement the change.

According to the PARiHS framework, if there is strong evidence, a receptive context, and effective facilitation, then successful implementation can be realized. However, if one or two of the three components are weak, the other(s) must be strong. Further explanation of the three major components of the equation is as follows. Evidence can be explained as codified or non-codified knowledge sources, which include research, experience, preferences, and local information. Context is related to aspects of the organization, such as networks, culture, and leadership. Some contexts are more conducive to change than others. Those would include contexts with transformational leaders, learning organizations, and those with appropriate monitoring and feedback channels.

The type of facilitation and role of the facilitator which is required are determined by the individuals and teams receiving this change, namely, their understanding of the evidence and level of receptiveness.[14] The PARiHS model is pertinent to this program because it has a focus on the organization, rather than on individuals. Within this program the Nurse Executive represents the organization and discipline of nursing as a whole.

## Change Model

The model that fits with this program is Roger's Diffusion Model. This model's major concepts are communication channels, characteristics of social systems, members, and innovation. There are five stages: knowledge, persuasion, decision, implementation, and confirmation. Roger's model is time-oriented, linear, and unidirectional. It spreads innovation over time and focuses attention on "persons as adopters."[23] Simply gaining new knowledge does not guarantee new practices or improved competencies. The translation of that knowledge into practice must occur, and for this an appropriate training model and appropriate methodologies are key.[28]

Roger's Diffusion Model is ideal for this setting. Germane to this program is the model's characteristic that adopters' needs must be at the core of the successful change, and that efforts are tailored to the local need. Thus, the Nurse Executive will support Roger's tenet of knowing the social system with the ability to see the situation from the perspective of potential adopters. In order to meet strategic goals, it is imperative that a self-assessment, and the subsequent adoption and incorporation of the newly gained knowledge and critical components into practice, are carried out.[29] A framework that supports incorporation over time of new training and competencies will lead to improved practice outcomes. This framework needs to be flexible and practical, and must allow for progression between categories.[22] Roger's Diffusion Model embodies these characteristics.

# Program Need and Supporting Evidence

This program is based on the development of a Nurse Executive Toolkit for Disaster Response. As this is a fairly new arena for health care practitioners, though one that has received considerable attention in recent years, it is incumbent on nurse leaders to ensure they are prepared to plan for and manage nursing care during a disaster. Disaster response has not historically been part of nursing curricula and thus little education and training has existed for the bulk of nurses in practice today.

Nurse Executives have the responsibility for developing a framework for care delivery during a disaster, which includes competent patient care and managing resources.[8] This responsibility also includes developing and delivering the necessary workplace training.[3] A toolkit to guide the Nurse Executive will be a valuable resource to address the complexities involved in competencies needed for disaster response. It is imperative that nursing at all levels be educated about their role and responsibilities within the organization and how they will be expected to function during a disaster.[6,9]

Keeping in mind that many nurses have little to no training in disaster response, especially those who were trained before the recent introduction of this subject into curricula, Nurse Executives also need assistance in this area. They may well be seasoned, experienced, and educated clinicians and administrators, but they have limited exposure to disaster response and the responsibilities and functions expected of them. The Nurse Executive will be expected to develop policies and plans that will result in effective and efficient nursing functions within their organization, even though applying competency-based education and training is a relatively new concept.[11]

## Program Description

Implementing the program in the Nurse Executive Toolkit for Disaster Response will result in actualization of prepared and trained nurse leaders in the acute care hospital setting. The initial phase will consist of a six-month planning period, followed by an initial implementation phase of six months. Those included are the Nurse Executive, Associate Nurse Executives, and an administrative assistant for clerical support. Also included, in keeping with Kitson's Model, is a facilitator for the group. The aforementioned personnel are consistent with the Roger's Diffusion Model tenet of knowing the social systems members and persons as adopters.

This group of Nurse Executives will meet twice monthly for six months. They will be charged with the responsibilities identified in the Nurse Executive competencies in this program plan, and with developing an implementation and evaluation plan. Within this schedule, the group should have the flexibility to decide to do a pilot or targeted, incremental implementation, depending on their particular needs. A program evaluation at six months and twelve months will be completed by the Nurse Executive, in order to provide an assessment of the toolkit plan.

The toolkit was designed to provide competencies identified as critical for the Nurse Executive and which are applicable to the scope and standards of practice for a nurse administrator.[2] In keeping with the measurement criteria for scope of practice and other recommendations in the literature for measuring competency outcomes, a list of competencies and measurement criteria for each has been formulated.[11,13,19,22] Nine competencies have been identified, which are categorized into three domains, listed in Table 2-1.

The toolkit will contain resources from the literature on current evidence-based practice recommendations. An established model for disaster nursing in the military, using the three-phase approach for pre-event, event, and post-event, will be the framework for the training model.[30] Additional resources included in the toolkit will include: guidelines for capability assessment, a resource list of other agencies (state and federal) which may interface with nursing personnel during a disaster, and standard triage guidelines. However, specific needs for the particular organization will be identified and developed by the Nurse Executive and team.[11]

## Goals/Aims

The goal of this program is for the Nurse Executive to accomplish the individual competencies as categorized in the three main domains (Table 2-1). This toolkit for Nurse Executives, which provides a basic framework that they can customize, can be used in their practice to achieve those competencies. Competencies for Nurse Executives who are in leadership positions are different than those for frontline staff, with a focus on organizational and strategic decision making, resource management, and policy.[4] Aims of this program are summarily described in the list of targeted functions, which are directly related to the competencies referenced in Table 2-1. These are based on needs assessment and current recommendations in the literature. The following goals/aims are summarily described in a Gantt Chart, found in Table 2-2.

List of Goals/Aims:

1. Identify key stakeholders involved in the program

    - Nurse Executives may identify other helpful and pertinent staff to participate, such as middle management staff or administrative officers

        - Key stakeholders can be defined as those in leadership or management positions who may be involved with or who can effectively address the criteria outlined in the Nurse Executive Competencies.

- Role assignments will be made by the end of month 1.

2. Review existing policies/plans and conduct capability assessment

- If no policy currently exists for nursing practice and functions during a disaster, one should be developed; existing policy should be reviewed and revised as applicable.

- A capability assessment can be accomplished using the toolkit guide; first draft to be submitted by end of month 2; a second assessment later may be beneficial.

3. Review resource management components

- Resource management is extensive in scope. Timeline for implementation of training model and surge capacity bed expansion will be finalized by the end of month 3.

4. Review professional practice components

- Procurement plans for needed resources will be finalized by end of month 5.

5. Draft policy

- Policy should include responsibilities and processes assigned for training, resources and nursing personnel functions. This can be a nursing policy or included as subsections in a broader hospital policy on disasters. Final draft will be completed by end of month 6.

6. Conduct evaluation

- Initial evaluation will be conducted at month 12 and at regular intervals thereafter.

## SWOT Analysis

The Strengths, Weaknesses, Opportunities, and Threats (SWOT) analysis is a method to evaluate strategic planning. The SWOT analysis is useful to identify both internal and external factors that may affect the program goals and objectives, either favorably or unfavorably. An explanation of the SWOT components is as follows. Strengths are organizational elements that may have positive effects; weaknesses are those that may have negative effects. Opportunities are external circumstances or influences that may be supportive to the program goals, and outcomes and threats are external factors that could be harmful. The SWOT analysis for this program is described in the Table 2-3. A sample budget is illustrated in Table 2-4.

## Summary

Developing and addressing Nurse Executive competencies for disaster response is a crucial and significant responsibility for a nurse leader. It requires a strategic plan and systematic approach that should compel stakeholder buy-in and adoption. The ultimate outcome will be the implementation of a program that will lead to enhanced nursing practice during a disaster. In addition, it will engage nursing leadership in a collaborative and proactive manner in addressing disaster response across the organization and how nursing integrates into that plan. It will require and promote a culture of open communication and innovation.

# Table 2-1
## Nurse Executive Competencies[5,11,12,19,22]

| Domain | Competency | Measurement Criteria |
|---|---|---|
| Administrative Leadership | 1. Policy Development | 1. Develop policy and procedure to address nursing training and practice for disaster response. |
| | 2. Incident Command | 2. Understand the incident command structure for your organization and how nursing integrates with that structure. |
| | 3. Capability Assessment | 3. Conduct a systematic capability assessment, based on your organization's structure and staffing, and identify gaps and vulnerabilities. |
| Resource Management | 1. Training Model | 1. Implement an evidence-based disaster response training model for nursing. |
| | 2. Surge Capacity Bed Expansion | 2. Develop a bed expansion plan, using your capability assessment and organizational disaster plan. |
| | 3. Systems Interoperability | 3. Identify how nursing interfaces with other disciplines, agencies, and organizations involved during a disaster, particularly regarding communication, information security, and lines of authority. |
| Professional Practice | 1. Triage and Patient Movement | 1. Incorporate standard triage model and recognize need for patient movement and tracking system in order to maximize efficiency of care during a disaster with mass casualties. |
| | 2. Altered Standards of Care | 2. Address altered standards of care, which may be necessary to maximize lives saved during a disaster with mass casualties. |
| | 3. Ethical and Psychological Issues | 3. Recognize ethical and psychological concerns that may arise during a disaster and identify resources for support. |

## Table 2-2
**Gantt Chart**

|  | Month 1 | 2 | 3 | 4 | 5 | 6 | 12 |
|---|---|---|---|---|---|---|---|
| Initial meeting: charter group, mission, assign roles, and identify points of contact for targeted tasks. *(Roger's Diffusion stage: Knowledge)* | X | | | | | | |
| Review existing plans/ policies; conduct capability assessment. | | X | | | | | |
| Identify timeline for implementation. Review resource management domain. *(Roger's Diffusion stage: Persuasion)* | | | X | | | | |
| Determine resources needed for professional practice components & make arrangements for procurement. | | | | X | | | |
| Draft policy. Assign specific evaluators for major sections/domains. *(Roger's Diffusion stage: Decision)* | | | | | X | | |
| Approve final draft of policy and schedule roll out. Review process for evaluation, including quantitative and qualitative tools. *(Roger's Diffusion stage: Implementation)* | | | | | | X | |
| Program Evaluation *(Roger's Diffusion stage: Confirmation)* | | | | | | | X |

## Table 2-3
### SWOT Analysis

| | |
|---|---|
| Strengths | - Not resource intensive<br>- Financially affordable<br>- Learning organization<br>- Culture of willingness to innovate |
| Weaknesses | - Requires personnel for planning and ongoing operations<br>- May be perceived as non-essential during times of staffing shortages<br>- May be difficult to find effective facilitator |
| Opportunities | - Increasing support for this type of preparation from regulatory bodies and professional and specialty organizations<br>- Evidence in the literature supports and recommends this type of program |
| Threats | - Competing activities and responsibilities may be a distraction<br>- Budgeting constraints may hamper effectiveness |

# Table 2-4
**Sample Budget**

|  | Initial Program Implementation | Program Evaluation at Month 12 |
|---|---|---|
| <u>Fixed Expenses</u> | | |
| Office Supplies | $ 225 | $ 75 |
| Printing/Media | 100 | 50 |
| Educational Material | 150 | 0 |
| | | |
| <u>Variable Expenses</u> | *Twelve one-hour sessions:* | *Three one-hour sessions:* |
| Nurse Executive @ $75/hour | $ 900 | $ 225 |
| Associate Nurse Executives, 4 @ $60/hour | 2,880 | 720 |
| Administrative Assistant @ $15/hour | 600 | 150 |
| Facilitator @ $30/hour | 1,440 | 360 |
| | | |
| <u>Staff work between meetings:</u> | | |
| -20 hours per month x 6 months @ $30/hour | 3,600 | |
| Sub Totals | 9,895 | 1,580 |
| Grand Total   $ 11,475 | | |

## References

1. Akins, R., Williams, J., Silenas, R. & Edwards, J. (2005). The role of public health nurses in bioterrorism preparedness. *Disaster Management and Response, 3,* 98-105.

2. American Nurses Association (2009). *Nursing administration scope and standards of practice.* Silver Spring, MD: Nursesbooks.org.

3. Boatright, C. & McGlown, K. (2005). Homeland security challenges in nursing practice. *Nursing Clinics of North America, 40,* 481-497.

4. Contino, D. (2004). Leadership competencies: Knowledge, skills and aptitudes nurses need to lead organizations effectively. *Critical Care Nurse, 24,* 52-64.

5. Danna, D., Bernard, M., Jones, J. & Matthews, P. (2009). Improvements in disaster planning and directions for nursing management. *The Journal of Nursing Administration, 39,* 423-431.

6. Drenkard, K., Rigotti, G., Hanfling, D., Fahlgren, T. & LaFrancois, G. (2002). Healthcare system disaster preparedness, part 1: planning. *The Journal of Nursing Administration, 32,* 461-469.

7. Encarta Dictionary. Retrieved November 24, 2009, from: http://uk.encarta.msn.com/encnet/features/dictionaryresults.aspx.

8. Fahlgren, T. & Drenkard, K. (2002). Healthcare system disaster preparedness, part 2: Nursing executive role in leadership. *The Journal of Nursing Administration, 32,* 531-537.

9. Gebbie, K. & Qureshi, K. (2002). Emergency and disaster preparedness. *American Journal of Nursing, 102,* 46-51.

10. Helitzer, D., Hollis, C., de Hernandez, B., Sanders, M., Roybal, S. & VanDeusen, I. (2009). Evaluation for community-based programs: The integration of logic models and factor analysis. *Evaluation and Program Planning, 10, 18-24.*

11. Hsu, E., Thomas, T., Bass, E., Whyne, D., Kelen, G. & Green, G. (2006). Healthcare worker competencies for disaster training. *BioMed Central Medical Education, 6,* 19.

12. Issel, L. (2004). *Health program planning and evaluation.* Sudbury, MA: Jones and Bartlett Publishers.

13. Jakeway, C., LaRosa, G. & Schoenfisch, S. (2008). The role of public health nurses in emergency preparedness and response: A position paper of the Association of State and Territorial Directors of Nursing. *Public Health Nursing, 25,* 323-361.

14. Kitson, A., Rycroft-Malone, J., Harvey, G., McCormack, B. & Seers, K. (2008). Evaluating the successful implementation of evidence into practice using the PARiHS framework. *BioMed Central Medical Education, 3.*

15. Lyznicki, J., Subbarao, I., Benjamin, G. & James, J. (2007). Developing a consensus framework for an effective and efficient disaster response health system: A national call to action. *Disaster Medicine and Public Health Preparedness, 1,* S51-54.

16. Markenson, D. DiMaggio, C. & Redlener, I. (2005). Preparing health professions students for terrorism, disaster, and public health emergencies: Core competencies. *Academic Medicine, 80,* 517-526.

17. Melynk, B. & Fineout-Overholt, E. (2005). *Evidence-based practice in nursing & healthcare.* Philadelphia, PA.: Lippincott, Williams & Wilkins.

18. Polivka, B., Stanley, S., Gordon, D. Taulbee, K., Kieffer, G. & McCorkle, S. (2008). Public health nursing competencies for public health surge events. *Public Health Nursing, 25,* 159-165.

19. Powers, R. & Daily, E. (2010). *International disaster nursing.* Cambridge, MA: Cambridge University Press.

20. Rebman, T. (2006). Defining bioterrorism preparedness for nurses: Concept analysis. *Journal of Advanced Nursing, 54,* 623-632.

21. Slepski, L. (2005). Emergency preparedness: Concept development for nursing practice. *Nursing Clinics of North America, 40,* 419-430.

22. Subbarao, I., Lyznicki, J., Hsu, E., Gebbie, K., Markenson, D., Barzansky, B., ... James, J. (2008). A consensus-based educational framework and competency set for the discipline of disaster medicine and public health preparedness. *Disaster Medicine and Public Health Preparedness, 2,* 57-68.

23. Tiffany, C. & Lutjens, L. (1998). *Planned change theories for nursing.* Thousand Oaks, CA: SAGE Publications.

24. Torghele, K., Buyum, A., Dubruiel, N., Augustine, J., Houlihan, C., Alperin, M. & Miner, K. (2007). Logic model use in developing a survey instrument for program evaluation: Emergency preparedness summits for schools of nursing in Georgia. *Public Health Nursing, 24,* 472-479.

25. Veenema, T. (2003). *Disaster nursing and emergency preparedness for chemical, biological and radiological terrorism and other hazards.* New York, NY: Springer Publishing Company.

26. *Webster's New College Dictionary*. (2008). Boston, MA: Houghton Mifflin Harcourt.

27. Weiner, E. (2005). A national curriculum for nurses in emergency preparedness and response. *Nursing Clinics of North America, 40,* 469-479.

28. Williams, J., Nocera, M. & Casteel, C. (2008). The effectiveness of disaster training for health care workers: A systematic review. *Annals of Emergency Medicine, 52,* 211-222.

29. Wisniewski, R., Dennik-Champion, G. & Peltier, J. (2004). Emergency preparedness competencies. The *Journal of Nursing Administration, 34,* 475-480.

30. Wynd, C. (2006). A proposed model for military disaster nursing. *The Online Journal of Issues in Nursing, 11*.

# Chapter 3

**Training Model**

# Introduction

Responding to a disaster, even when well prepared, can be overwhelming. It forces clinicians outside of their comfort zones and requires delivery of care in stressful, and sometimes austere and dangerous situations. It is therefore imperative to be as prepared as possible. Training that is realistic, relative, and timely supports that preparation. Nurse Executives should evaluate and plan for training in their facilities that is relative to nursing practice. A training model that is useful for nurses is described herein.

# Practice

The goal of this training model is not to produce experts or provide extensive, in-depth academic education, but rather to provide a basic framework from which Nurse Executives can design or customize training for their nursing staff which will give them basic knowledge and skills for disaster response. The use of evidence-based education is desirable. It is widely recognized that the military has extensive experience in this field and that much of the knowledge, research, and lessons learned can be applied to civilian practice.[1,6] Therefore, this training model is based largely on the three-phase approach used for military nursing. Those three phases as described by Jennings-Sanders[3] are as follows:

1. Preparedness and readiness
2. Response and implementation
3. Recovery, reconstruction, and evaluation

Effective methods for training are just as important as the model. A combination of modalities is recommended. "Hands-on" training and drills cannot be overemphasized. These are essential for gaining a realistic experience and help staff gain needed skills with equipment, communication methods, and protocols for patient processing.[4,6] Another training component is the learning module, such as those available from government entities, including the Federal Emergency Management Agency, Centers for Disease Control, or other academic institutions or agencies which have produced web-based training.[2,4] The advantage of this type of training module is that it can be done in any location with computer and Internet access as a self-learning opportunity, as well as in a group setting for larger numbers of staff. In addition, another recommended training opportunity is the table top exercise. For those situations where a full-scale drill is not feasible, a table top exercise can be beneficial, especially for some of the more administrative aspects, such as command center functions, pre-hospital activity, and logistical elements of patient movement.[2,5] A table top exercise is conducted sitting around a table, discussing and reviewing a scenario, rather than doing a "hands-on" episode in the field.

A more academic approach to disaster response preparedness and training is that of utilizing research and literature. Holding regular journal clubs or conferences with review and discussion of current literature can be very beneficial in gaining knowledge about disaster response.[4] In addition, conducting research specific to nursing can be an engaging and skill-building experience. Designing a local research project or submitting research questions to other bodies will assist nursing staff in identifying training needs, as well as developing a mindset of using scientific and evidence-based approaches to improving practice.[1,6]

Nurse Executives can use this three-phase training model as a framework and then customize it to the specific needs of their facility and staff. Use of specific training modalities, especially full disaster drills, will likely depend on local policy, availability, and financial feasibility. However, with such a variety of training opportunities available, especially no-cost, web-based modules, an effective three-phase training model can be realized. An outline of that model is described in Table 3-1.

# Table 3-1
## Three-Phase Training Model

| Phase | Actions |
|---|---|
| 1. Preparedness | • Establish competencies<br>• Training for:<br>  ➢ Disaster plans<br>  ➢ Clinical skills<br>    ▪ Equipment, personal protective gear, decontamination, types of potential injuries<br>  ➢ Triage<br>  ➢ Command center functions<br>  ➢ Communication<br>  ➢ Bed expansion and surge capacity<br>  ➢ Patient movement<br>  ➢ Networking with other community agencies<br>• Psychological and ethical considerations |
| 2. Response | • Implement disaster plans<br>• Provide care for casualties |
| 3. Recovery | • Evaluation of disaster response<br>  ➢ Write after action reports within thirty days of the conclusion of the disaster<br>• Identify strengths and weakness of response<br>  ➢ plans for corrective actions, including additional training<br>• Debrief staff involved in disaster<br>  ➢ Evaluation of event and response<br>  ➢ Self-evaluations<br>  ➢ Identify psychological needs<br>• Staff recognition<br>• Recovery of supplies and equipment |

## References

1. Bridges, E., Schmelz, J. & Kellkey, P. (2008). Military nursing research: Translation to disaster response and day to day critical care nursing. *Critical Care Nursing Clinics of North America, 20*, 121-131.

2. Dembek, Z., Iton, A. & Hansen, H. (2005). A model curriculum for public health bioterrorism education. *Public Health Reports, 120*, 11-18.

3. Jennings-Sanders, A. (2004). Teaching disaster nursing by utilizing the Jennings Disaster Nursing Management model. *Nursing Education in Practice, 4*, 69-76.

4. Koenig, K., Bey, T. & Schultz, C. (2009). International disaster medical sciences fellowship: Model curriculum and key considerations for establishment of an innovative international educational program. *Western Journal of Emergency Medicine, 4*, 213-219.

5. Lee, W., Kuan, J., Shiau, Y., Chen, C., Ng, C., Chiu, T. & Chen, J. (2003). Designation of a new training model of a local disaster medical system with tabletop exercises. *Chang Gung Medical Journal, 12*, 879-888.

6. Wynd, C. (2006). A proposed model for military disaster nursing. *Online Journal of Issues in Nursing, 11*.

# Chapter 4

**Triage**

## Background

During disasters with large-scale mass casualties, triage is an essential component in efficiently treating and processing victims. Outside the disaster response realm, triage can have a variety of meanings and definitions depending on the setting. However, during a disaster, it is important that a systematic and standard approach to triage be taken and understood by all parties involved. During a disaster, resources are often scarce and disaster response personnel have ethical and legal responsibilities to use those resources responsibly.[3] Effective triage aims to provide the best survivability to the greatest number. Field triage of casualties is the first step in matching a patient with the services and level of care needed.[6] Since many levels of personnel and disciplines will interface during a disaster, it is imperative that an interoperable understanding of triage exist.[2]

## Practice

For the Nurse Executive planning nursing care during a disaster response, understanding the triage categories of patients arriving will be integral to effectively treating those casualties. The pre-hospital triage system typically used by both civilian and military responders is a color-coded system as explained herein.

The START (Simple Triage and Rapid Treatment) system was developed in California by a hospital system and fire department. It was designed to assess a patient quickly in less than a minute. A tag is attached to the patient with the applicable triage designation. The patient is then treated by rescue or responder personnel as the triage officer quickly moves on to triage other victims. This system is designed to provide the best chance to save as many patients as possible. The colored tags have the following designations.[4]

Green = Minor: walking wounded, care can be delayed several hours

Yellow = Delayed: needs are urgent, but care can be delayed up to an hour

Red = Immediate: life-threatening injuries, needs care immediately

Black = Deceased

The military model also uses a color-coded system, with only slightly different terminology.

Green = Minimal: walking wounded

Yellow = Delayed: requires care within six hours

Red = Immediate: needs immediate care for potential fatal injuries

Black = Expectant: dead or dying, not expected to reach a higher level of care alive; treat after other categories of patients have been treated

The order in which these categories of patients are treated is immediate, delayed, minimal and expectant.[1]

Triage is a dynamic process and the patient should be reassessed at each level of care. Once patients arrive at the hospital, they will be re-triaged based on their current condition, as it may have changed from the time they were initially triaged in the field. Hospital triage may be conducted differently than pre-hospital or field triage, but it is important for hospital personnel to be familiar with field hospital triage, in order to understand the categories and conditions of patients being received from the field.

## Sample Triage Tag

| TRIAGE TAG |
| :---: |
| No: 123456 |

Major Injuries

| Time | BP | Pulse | Resp | Prescription Meds |
|---|---|---|---|---|
|  |  |  |  |  |
|  |  |  |  |  |
|  |  |  |  | Allergies |
|  |  |  |  |  |

Personal Information

Name_____   Male   Female
Address_____
City/State_____   Age_____
Phone_____   Weight_____

Emergency Contact_____

**Hospital Destination:**

Notes:

| **DECEASED** |
| :---: |
| No: 123456 |

| **IMMEDIATE** | | |
| :--- | :---: | ---: |
| No: 123456 | *Life Threatening* | Priority 1 |

| **DELAYED** | | |
| :--- | :---: | ---: |
| No: 123456 | *Serious, Non-Life Threatening* | Priority 2 |

| **MINOR** | | |
| :--- | :---: | ---: |
| No: 123456 | *Walking Wounded* | Priority 3 |

# References

1. Army Study Guide (2005). Retrieved January 28, 2011 from: http://www.armystudyguide.com/content/powerpoint/First_Aid_Presentations/triage-2.shtml.

2. Bostick, N., Subbarao, I., Burkle, F., Hsu, E., Armstrong, J. & James, J. (2008). Disaster triage systems for large-scale catastrophic events. *Disaster Medicine and Public Health Preparedness,* 2 (Suppl 1: S35–S39).

3. Larkin, G. & Arnold, J. (2003). Ethical considerations in emergency planning, preparedness, and response to acts of terrorism. *Prehospital and Disaster Medicine,* 18:170–178.

4. Start Triage (2011). Retrieved January 28, 2011 from: http://www.start-triage.com.

5. Zoraster, R., Chidester, C. & Koenig, W. (2007). Field triage and patient maldistribution in a mass-casualty incident. *Prehospital and Disaster Medicine,* 22(3):224–229.

# Chapter 5

**Capability Assessment**

## Introduction

Being prepared for a disaster is crucial to successful management of a large influx of casualties. Several factors affect being prepared: utilizing a checklist for planning is one method for systematic assessment, mitigation, and response. Strategies include a comprehensive knowledge of your facility disaster plan, as well as specific administrative skills as the Nurse Executive, who is key to quickly mobilizing and managing nursing care during a disaster.

## Concepts and Strategies

For the Nurse Executive to conduct a capability assessment, the major concepts to be addressed can be outlined in these categories:

- staff
- space
- supplies
- communication
- patient movement

One strategy for using a checklist is that it will help identify areas of weakness which may need some additional planning or attention, or further discussion about how the facility can address or support aspects of nursing care delivery during a disaster. An adequate supply is defined as a supply for three to five days, as this is the usual amount of time expected for outside help to arrive. A capability assessment checklist has been developed after analyzing and synthesizing examples and recommendations from entities listed as references in this document. The checklist is listed as Table 5-1.

## Table 5-1
### Capability Assessment Checklist

| Concept | Assessment criteria | Comments |
|---|---|---|
| Staff | • Recall roster with contact information for all staff members<br><br>• Process in place to activate recall or emergency call in for staff<br><br>• Designated point of contact or coordinator to initiate recall<br><br>• Defined roles or actions for staff during disaster<br><br>• Designated point of assembly or staging area for staff responding to disaster recall<br><br>• Registration and assignment process for staff responding to disaster recall<br><br>• Parking issues<br><br>• Protocol for tiered or staggered staffing to cover all shifts with limited staff who may get only intermittent rest periods<br><br>• Protocol for housing staff if they cannot leave facility<br><br>• Process for just in time training for specific disaster needs<br><br>• Resources available for specific patient care needs during disaster (i.e., biological exposure, blast injuries, burns, etc.)<br><br>• Drills, training, or competency verification for staff<br><br>• Staff understands command center structure and chain of command<br><br>• Labor issues: overtime, can't report to work, hazardous duty<br><br>• Process for demobilizing staff when disaster is over or relief help arrives<br><br>• Staff debriefing and potential counseling needs after disaster is over | |

| Concept | Assessment criteria | Comments |
|---|---|---|
| **Supplies** | • Supply or cache of particular items specially designated for a disaster and, if so, nursing staff knows how to access it | |
| | • Facility disaster plan with provision for adequate supply of personal protective equipment | |
| | • Process for supplying hand sanitizer or alternate hand washing methods if regular sinks or hand washing methods are not available | |
| | • Extra beds, stretchers, or cots for use with surge capacity in a disaster and, if so, designation of where they are kept and who will retrieve them | |
| | • Adequate supply of equipment such as IV pumps and poles, ventilators, and suction machines; designation of who is responsible for managing this inventory | |
| | • Adequate supply of medications available from pharmacy | |
| | • Adequate supply and a process for sterilizing surgical equipment or disposable equipment | |
| | • Linen supplies: an adequate supply; process for obtaining fresh supply if the facility does not have the ability to process its own linen | |
| | • Supplies for processing and handling potentially contaminated specimens (such as with biological or chemical exposures), and, if so, nursing staff knows how to access them | |
| | • Protocol for supply rationing or prioritization of use if adequate supplies are not readily available | |
| | • Adequate supply of paper forms in the event electronic documentation systems go down | |

| Concept | Assessment criteria | Comments |
|---|---|---|
| **Space** | • Plan for extra bed set-up for surge capacity, utilizing space not typically used: hallways, clinics, waiting rooms, therapy rooms, or plan for bed expansion in existing patient rooms<br><br>• Areas designated for families and visitors in addition to the usual waiting rooms (which may be taken for other uses)<br><br>• Nursing staff is aware of potential space use modifications and conversion in the event of a disaster and knows where to locate specific functions and operations if they are in an alternate location<br><br>• Specific rooms or space designated for isolation or decontamination<br><br>• Signage available to label rooms designated for alternative use | |

| Concept | Assessment criteria | Comments |
|---|---|---|
| Communication | • There is a plan for using radios, a messenger, or runners in the event regular communication systems go down<br><br>• There is a plan for communication methods if electricity and power are lost<br><br>• Nursing personnel has access to portable, wireless computers, cell phones, or radios and plans for extras to be obtained on short notice for use in a large scale disaster<br><br>• There is a plan for how orders and diagnostic test results will be communicated between ancillary departments and caregivers in the absence of an electronic medical record<br><br>• Nursing staff is familiar with the command center process for communication, i.e., overhead announcements, radio use, or internal TV channel messaging<br><br>• Nursing staff is aware of or has guidelines for what communication may be required with outside agencies<br><br>• Specific personnel is designated to be the official spokesperson to outside agencies and organizations | |

| Concept | Assessment criteria | Comments |
|---|---|---|
| **Patient Movement** | • Routes for patient movement are clearly identified for a large influx of patients (access and egress routes)<br><br>• There are traffic flow maps available<br><br>• There is a specific receiving, staging, and triage area or alternate plan for all casualties to process through the emergency department<br><br>• Nursing staff is familiar with standard triage tags assigned to patients in the field or pre-hospital<br><br>• Plans are in place to quickly identify and process patients who can be discharged or moved to a different level of care<br><br>• There is a process for cancellation of elective or non-emergency surgeries and procedures<br><br>• Plans to restrict or control elevator use<br><br>• Designation of personnel and resources are available for patient transport<br><br>• If there are satellite locations where some casualties will be housed or treated, there is a plan for how they get there<br><br>• There are areas designated for refuge in the event there is an in-hospital emergency or evacuation is necessary<br><br>• Plan for how patient records and documents are transported or moved from one location to another with the patient<br><br>• Plan for how patient movement is tracked:<br><br>• throughout the hospital<br><br>• in the event the patient is transferred to another facility | |

## Bibliography

1. *American Health Lawyers Association*. Retrieved December 18, 2010 from: http://www.healthlawyers.org/Resources/PI/InfoSeries/Documents/Emergency%20Preparedness%20Checklist.pdf.

2. *Association for Professionals in Infection Control and Epidemiology*. Retrieved February 4, 2011 from: http://www.apic.org/bioterror/checklist.doc.

3. Austin, B., Allswede, M., Cantrill, S. & Bravata, D. (2003). Optimizing surge capacity: Hospital assessment and planning. *Agency for Healthcare Research and Quality*. Retrieved December 19, 2010 from: http://archive.ahrq.gov/news/ulp/bt-briefs/btbrief3.htm.

4. Belmont, E., Fried, B., Gonen, J., Murphy, A., Sconyers, J. & Zinder, S. (2004). Emergency preparedness, response and recovery checklist: Beyond the emergency management plan. *Journal of Health Law, 37,* 503-565.

5. Centers for Disease Control (2011). Managing surge needs for injuries: Administration response. Retrieved February 4, 2011 from: http://www.bt.cdc.gov/masscasualties/pdf/Administration Response-508.pdf.

6. Centers for Disease Control (2011). Managing surge needs for injuries: Nursing care. Retrieved February 4, 2011 from: http://www.bt.cdc.gov/masscasualties/pdf/Nursing_Care-508.pdf.

# Chapter 6

**Program Evaluation**

In order to assess the effectiveness of the disaster response training program, an evaluation tool has been included in the toolkit. The Nurse Executive and leadership team can use this for the initial and annual evaluations to identify areas for improvement or additional needs. A qualitative evaluation may be accomplished by using the Strength, Weakness, Opportunity, and Threat (SWOT) analysis (Table 6-1). A quantitative evaluation can be accomplished with an evaluation checklist (Table 6-2). Both are included in this toolkit and either can be used, based on the preference of the Nurse Executive.

## Table 6-1
**Program SWOT Analysis**

| Strengths | • Identify aspects of this plan that have worked well: |
|---|---|
| Weaknesses | • Identify disadvantages, weaknesses, or areas for improvement: |
| Opportunities | • Identify new or revised tactics or innovations: |
| Threats | • Identify obstacles and organizational constraints: |

Additional information or resources you would find beneficial:

# Table 6-2
## Program Evaluation Checklist

Use the following rating scale to evaluate the program components in meeting your needs.

1. Not helpful

2. Somewhat helpful

3. Very helpful

| Component | Assessment Rating | | | Comments |
|---|---|---|---|---|
| Nurse Executive Competencies | 1 | 2 | 3 | |
| Triage Model | 1 | 2 | 3 | |
| Training Model | 1 | 2 | 3 | |
| Capability Assessment | 1 | 2 | 3 | |
| Agency and Resources List | 1 | 2 | 3 | |
| Overall Program Plan | 1 | 2 | 3 | |

Total Score _____

Additional information or resources you would find beneficial:

# Chapter 7

**Quality of Care Degradation during Disasters:
Practice Implications and Ethical Dilemmas**

# Introduction

Delivering medical care during disaster response requires deviations from routine practice. This chapter reviews the literature on changes in quality of care, practice and methods of care delivery, and the ethical concerns associated with disaster response health care. Practice which normally focuses on providing the highest standard of care for the individual becomes altered during disaster response, moving to the principle of the greatest good for the greatest number. A number of ethical dilemmas can arise from how decisions are made, rationing of care and supplies, and legal issues, as well as from short- and long-term impact on patients and health care workers.

# Background

In the last ten years, the number and magnitude of disasters resulting in mass casualties have been staggering. The terrorist attacks on the United States in September 2001 were jarring events that awakened the medical community to the crucial need for better preparation for handling such situations. Subsequent events, both man-made and natural, have reinforced the concerns of health care providers worldwide about providing care for mass casualties. Within our own borders we've experienced hurricanes, flooding, and tornadoes that resulted in large-scale destruction affecting thousands. Internationally, there have been earthquakes, tsunamis, flooding, volcanic eruptions, and wars, also resulting in a staggering number of casualties. One has only to turn on the television or listen to the news to see how quickly the health care systems and providers become overwhelmed, emphasizing the need for adequate preparation and for the realization that practice and quality standards which we use under everyday circumstances will not be applicable or effective during disasters. This chapter will examine how practice is affected and the ethical dilemmas that can arise related to care delivery during disasters.

# Practice Implications

The Agency for Healthcare Research and Quality (AHRQ) convened a summit in 2004 to discuss how care standards may be impacted when dealing with mass casualties and what was needed to plan for such situations. Among their key findings were that disaster response would require an altered standard in order to save as many lives as possible and that resource allocation should be "fair and clinically sound," with a process that was transparent.[1] The "greatest good for the greatest number" principle, an essential tenet in disaster response, is divergent from the usual practice standard of the "highest standard of care for each individual," to which we are accustomed.[1,23]

## Vignettes from Recent Disasters

To illustrate actual experiences of health care providers, the following vignettes recount some recent disasters. During Hurricane Katrina, the city of New Orleans became the site of dire conditions. Massive flooding took out electrical power, roads, and bridges. At one medical center, the staff was stranded for several days with no power, water, or functional toilets. Compounding this was the fact that part of the building was flooded and the temperature was over $100^0$ F. Additional people from the surrounding community had converged on the medical center seeking refuge, so the infrastructure was overwhelmed. Patients were evacuated from unsafe or flooded areas to other locations. Some patients could not be physically moved by the staff due to their conditions. They tried to take the patients to the garage so they could get to the helipad. After some time, realizing that no outside help was coming, private boats were arranged to help with the evacuation. All of this was being done in the dark and in sweltering heat. Medication administration and charting were problematic and some of the staff likened the circumstances to battlefield conditions.[19]

Severe storms in Australia in 2007 resulted in similar conditions with massive flooding, wind damage, destruction of roads, no electricity, no heat, dysfunctional sewage systems, and difficulty with preparing food. Emergency care at evacuation centers was challenging due to disruption in medication supplies, lack of power, and health threats from contaminated water. Injuries and conditions seen for treatment included hypothermia, fractures, lacerations, and gastroenteritis.[6]

Haiti experienced widespread, severe damage when a massive earthquake struck in 2010. Many buildings were completely flattened, or damaged beyond being habitable, so massive numbers of people were literally in the streets. Many were injured and scores more were buried beneath rubble. An Israeli medical team arrived in the country soon after the quake and set up a field hospital. They found a lack of coordination of medical care and resources. Their capability was quickly outpaced by the number of casualties, so they expanded bed capacity and added another table for surgery. They had to implement a triage system, which resulted in some patients being denied treatment. Because their capacity had reached its limit, they were forced to use a "one-to-one exchange" for patients, basically limiting receiving a new patient until one was able to leave. This team consisted of highly trained personnel who were prepared for such conditions, and yet even they were overwhelmed with casualties. Their facility was at its capacity within two days.[15,16] The United States Navy sent one of its hospital ships, the *Comfort*, to Haiti to assist in treating the mass casualties. Because they could provide tertiary care, critical patients were brought to the ship by helicopter. The challenges they faced were an extremely high number of casualties, patients who arrived with no medical history, and patients with multiple problems, not all of which could be addressed due to concentration on life-threatening conditions. An additional challenge was difficult discharge planning due to the nearly complete destruction of the Haitian medical system. Medical conditions included many fractures, crush injuries with renal failure, and infected wounds, some of which had worms and maggots.[2]

In the aftermath of the 2011 earthquake and subsequent tsunami in Japan widespread destruction resulted in thousands missing, dead, and injured. Hospitals were overwhelmed, ran out of food, had flooding in their own buildings, and operated with no water, electricity, or heat, while temperatures dropped to near freezing. One particular hospital sustained damage of equipment and part of its ceiling collapsed. Because the food and medication supplies were kept on the ground floor, when the lower levels were flooded, those supplies were damaged or destroyed. They were short on food and medicine and nurses resorted to trying to salvage what they could by cleaning muddy packages of intravenous fluids and pills with alcohol. They found some frozen noodles from a damaged freezer. The linen supply ran short and there weren't enough blankets.[5]

When a massive tornado struck Missouri in 2011, the city of Joplin was partially destroyed and the hospital heavily damaged. Patients had to be evacuated under dangerous conditions which included a fire in part of the hospital, broken windows, collapsed walls, debris and their damaged helicopter which had toppled into the parking lot. The staff made a remarkable evacuation of this 367 bed facility in ninety minutes and then set up a triage center in the parking lot. Unfortunately, there were five ventilator patients who died as a result of loss of power and the loss of their emergency generator, when it was blown away in the tornado. Medical records and other information, including x-rays were found miles away.[5]

A recurring theme in all these vignettes was the overwhelming volume of casualties and that care was focused on treating as many people as possible, triaging them based on the severity of their injuries and likelihood of survival. Even those individuals with multiple problems could not have all their problems addressed because the system and resources were outstripped by the sheer number of casualties. Some were turned away and received no treatment. This is a clear deviation from normal practice when we try to provide the highest quality of care for every patient and to address all their needs.

## Variations in Practice Standards

The AHRQ summit addressed this and developed a set of applicable standards as to what, to whom, when, by whom, and where care is given. It further discussed specific decisions that may have to be made regarding decreased standards. Some of those were: triage categories, possible reuse of supplies and equipment, resource distribution and rationing, documentation, privacy regulations, scope of practice, delays in care, processing fatalities, property seizures, and quarantine or mass immunizations. The AHRQ also developed a set of principles to serve as a framework for managing mass casualties. These are: to keep the system functioning to deliver acceptable quality of care to preserve as many lives as possible; have an adequate legal framework; have comprehensive, community-based planning, coordinated at the regional level; protect individual rights as much as possible and as is reasonable; provide clear communication with the public.[1]

Specific practice scenarios may include a variety of practice deviations, such as rationing of supplies and equipment, using triage categories, changing work conditions and locations, determining staffing availability and ratios, and functioning when the system is overwhelmed with casualties. One standard that should be maximized at all times is the safety of patient and health care worker[9] The AHRQ summit identified several steps for protecting health care providers: protective gear, training, staff rotation, mental health support, freedom from legal threats of malpractice, and support for providers' families.[1] In order to assess and improve quality standards, after an event, those who participated should objectively examine the event and the response and identify what improvements could be made.[9]

Rationing of supplies, staff, and equipment is a foreign concept to many of us. The thought that there may not be enough medical equipment, supplies, or medication is not the normal course of operations. However, during disasters, this will be necessary. Perhaps one of the most controversial pieces of equipment to be rationed may be ventilators, which will likely be reserved for those who have the best chance for survival. Protective gear for workers may also have to be rationed. Beds and services, and in particular specialty care, will be rationed. Diagnostic capabilities may have to be curtailed due to equipment availability.[10,13,14,21,23] Work conditions and locations will be affected. As illustrated in the vignettes of real disasters, staff found themselves working in damaged, flooded buildings with no services or in makeshift field conditions with evacuees. Communication and coordination of care will be impacted with the loss of regular telephone and cellular phone service. Radio communication can be hampered if the various medical centers, responders, and officials are using different systems.[12] Transporting patients during a disaster may be impacted, either by a lack of vehicles or by road closure or damage.[1] Another practice implication during disaster is that of working with volunteer staff who mobilize for care of mass casualties. Role definition and credentials verification may be a challenge. Setting priorities for patient care will involve an altered way of assessing and triaging patients. Battlefield triage may result in some patients, either those who have only minor injuries or those whose injuries are so serious that recovery is unlikely, being excluded from receiving care. The way in which patients are identified for discharge from a hospital in order to make room for a surge of casualties will function differently from the discharge process usually used.[9] When the health system is overwhelmed, there may be a breakdown in communication, both between health care facilities and with the public; ineffective interface between agencies; inefficient decision-making and coordination; lack of resources and personnel; and near panic by the public. All of these will negatively impact both the practicing health care worker and their patients.

## Ethical Dilemmas

It is widely recognized that dealing with mass casualties in disaster response raises legal and ethical questions, such as how resources are allocated, how this is communicated with stakeholders and the public, how the rights of the individual mesh with rights of society as a group, what the responsibilities of health care workers are, what the legal implications for health care workers are, what the long-term impacts on patients' health are, whether there is transparency with disaster policies and whether there is an accountability mechanism. In 2006, a summit was convened in Washington, D.C., during which experts in public health law, ethics, and practice were charged with developing principles for practice.[3]

The four basic ethical principles of beneficence, non-maleficence, autonomy, and justice have been around for some time[4] Additional ethical principles have been developed. One such set of principles features the following: duty to care, duty to steward resources, duty to plan, distributive justice, and transparency. Duty to care involves the precept of an "ethically sound rationing system." Duty to steward resources involves balancing obligations to each patient against the obligation to the entire community of patients. Duty to plan obligates authorities to develop guidelines prior to a disaster, acknowledging that it will not be perfect. Distributive justice requires that any allocation system must have consistent and broad application. Transparency involves making these guidelines available to the public and seeking public input.[21] The

2006 summit mentioned previously developed ten principles, divided into three categories, to address resource allocation in disasters.[3] They are depicted in Table 7-11.

Just as there are clinical triage protocols for patient conditions, resource triage exists as well. These guidelines for decision making should be objective, transparent, and involve key stakeholders in their development. Community discussions and education about how to use resources during mass casualties should help decrease some of the questions and problems of resource allocation. Triage scoring tools are being developed. One such tool is the Sequential Organ Failure Assessment (SOFA), which gives a numeric score. However, caution is recommended in using only a score to make such determinations.[20] It is advisable to have decisions regarding resource distribution made at a systems level and leave the clinical decisions about individual patients, utilizing the allocated resources, to the clinician. Once again, it is reinforced that a utilitarian construct of greatest good for the greatest number will become the norm in disaster situations.[9] As can be imagined, rationing of supplies and care would generate questions, aversion, and suspicion from a public that was not informed about or involved in planning and decision making. Therefore it is imperative that decisions be transparent and that some mechanism for accountability be present.

Unfortunately, these suspicions and questions, coupled with extremely stressful and calamitous conditions during a disaster, can lead to legal issues. The public will question whether everything was done that could have been done, why the system failed, why no help arrived sooner, how decisions were made, whether care was withheld unfairly, and whether some health care workers committed malpractice. One such situation was the arrest of a physician and two nurses in New Orleans who were accused of euthanizing patients at a medical center where they and the patients were stranded in the aftermath of Hurricane Katrina. The charges were denied by the workers and the grand jury refused to indict. The physician stated that she did give medication to the patients in question, as part of "comfort care," but not to kill them.[9,19] The fact that such charges and arrests would occur was shocking.

Impact of decreased quality standards on both patients and staff can be expected. One study highlighted the effect a disaster had on diabetic patients. Results demonstrated a negative effect on diabetic management and reduction in quality of life and life expectancy. Existing health care disparities were worsened by the disaster.[8] Health care workers are affected as well. They experience ethical and moral conflicts about decreased care standards, rationing of care, and making decisions they know will have negative consequences for individual patients.[9,16] Health care workers also encounter ethical conflicts about their duty to work. Conflicts include fear of personal injury or illness and worrying about familial responsibilities, versus their professional obligations to both their patients and their colleagues.[7,22] Patients and staff alike may suffer psychological effects from a disaster, either from the magnitude and trauma of the disaster itself, or from the ethical conflicts encountered. One study illustrated a higher level of stress in nurses who had treated war victims.[11] Post-traumatic stress related to war and other disasters has become a more visible topic in recent years and the psychological impact of disasters cannot be underestimated. By some accounts, up to ten percent of people who receive crisis counseling after an event are actually referred for professional mental health services.

## Summary

Mass casualties during disaster response can quickly overwhelm the health care system, requiring a reduction in quality standards that we pride ourselves on providing in everyday practice. It is widely recognized that this will be a requirement to try to meet the needs of the community as a whole. There is no doubt about the potential negative effects this may have on individual patients, communities, and the health care worker. An ethical framework and guidelines have been developed to assist in dealing with very difficult decisions made during disasters about changes in practice standards and the rationing or denial of care. Long-term physical and psychological effects can occur in patients and workers, but with more prominent recognition and plans for treatment, these effects can be mitigated. Broad discussions with community stakeholders are crucial for managing preparation for and managing the acute response and aftermath of disasters, in order to attain the most optimal outcomes.

# Table 7-11
## Ten Principles to Guide Resource Allocation[3]

| Category | Principle |
|---|---|
| Obligations to community | • Maintain transparency<br>• Conduct public health education and outreach |
| Balancing personal autonomy and community well-being/benefit | • Balance individual and communal needs to maximize the public health benefits of the populations being served while respecting individual rights, including providing mitigation for such infringements<br>• Consider the public health needs of individuals or groups without regard for their human condition |
| Good preparedness practice | • Adhere to and communicate applicable standard of care guidelines, absent an express directive by a governmental authority that suggests adherence to differing standards<br>• Identify public health priorities based on modern, scientifically sound evidence that supports the provision of resources to identified people<br>• Implement, in a prioritized, coordinated fashion, initiatives that are well-targeted to accomplishing essential public health services and core public health functions<br>• Assess the public health outcomes following a specific allocation decision, acknowledging that the process is iterative<br>• Ensure accountability pertaining to the specific duties and liabilities of people in the execution of the allocation decision<br>• Share personally identifiable health information—with the patients' consent where possible—solely to promote the health or safety of patients and other people |

## References

1. *Altered Standards of Care in Mass Casualty Events.* (2005). Agency for Healthcare Research and Quality, Publication No. 05-0043.

2. Amundson, D., Dadekian, G., Etienne, M., Gleeson, T., Hicke, T., Killiam, D., ... Miller, E. (2010). Practicing internal medicine onboard the USNS COMFORT in the aftermath of the Haitian earthquake. *Annals of Internal Medicine, 152*, 733-737.

3. Barnett, D., Taylor, H., Hodge, J. & Links, J. (2009). Resource allocation on the frontlines of public health preparedness and response: report of a summit on legal and ethical issues. *Public Health Reports, 124*, 295-303.

4. Beauchamp, T. & Childress, J. (2000). Principles of biomedical ethics. Oxford, Oxford University Press.

5. CBS News. Retrieved June 16, 2011 from: http://www.cbsnews.com/stories/2011/05/24/earlyshow/main20065622.shtml).

6. Cretikos, M., Merritt, T., Main, K, Eastwood, K., Winn, L. Moran, L. & Durrheim, D. (2007). Mitigating the health impacts of a natural disaster—the June 2007 long weekend storm in the Hunter region of New South Wales. *Medical Journal of Australia, 187*, 670-673.

7. Dodgen, D., Norwood, A., Becker, S., Perez, J. & Hansen, C. (2100). Social, psychological and behavioral responses to a nuclear detonation in a US city: implications for health care planning and delivery. *Disaster Medicine and Public Health Preparedness, 5*, (Suppl 1): S54-S64.

8. Fonseca, V., Smith, H., Kuhadiya, N., Leger, S., Yau, L., Reynolds, K., ... John-Kalarickal, J. (2009). Impact of a natural disaster on diabetes. *Diabetes Care, 32*, 1632-1638.

9. Gebbie, K., Peterson, C., Subbarao, I. & White, K. (2009). Adapting standards of care under extreme conditions. *Disaster Medicine and Public Health Preparedness, 3*, 111-116.

10. James, J., Benjamin, G., Burkle, F., Gebbie, K., Gabor, L. & Subbarao, I. (2010). Disaster medicine and public health preparedness: a discipline for all health professionals. *Disaster Medicine and Public Health Preparedness*, 4, 102-124.

11. Jayawardene, W., Youssef Agha, A., LaJoie, S. & Torabi, M. (2011). Psychological distress among nurses caring for victims of war in Sri Lanka. *Disaster Medicine and Public Health Preparedness, 5*, (doi:10.1001/dmp.2011.36), E1-E8.

12. Kahn, L. & Barondess, J. (2008). Preparing for disaster: response matrices in the USA and UK. *Journal of Urban Health, 85*, 910-922.

13. Kanter, R. & Moran, J. (2007). Hospital emergency surge capacity: an empiric New York statewide study. *Annals of Emergency Medicine, 50*, 314-319.

14. Koenig, K., Cone, D., Burstein, J. & Camargo, C. (2006). Surging to the right standard of care. *Society for Academic Emergency Medicine, 13*, 195-197.

15. Kreiss, Y., Merin, O., Peleg, K., Levy, G., Vinker, S., Sagi, R., ... Ash, N. (2010). Early disaster response in Haiti: the Israeli field hospital experience. *Annals of Internal Medicine, 153*, 45-48.

16. Merin, O., Ash, N., Levy, G., Schwaber, M. & Kreiss, Y. (2010). The Israeli field hospital in Haiti: ethical dilemmas in early disaster response. *New England Journal of Medicine, 362*, e38.

17. Misery at Japan's tsunami-ravaged hospitals (2011). Retrieved June 16, 2011 from: http://www.cbsnews.com/stories/2011/03/14/501364/main20042841.html.

18. Murphy, K. (2011). Five patients who died in Joplin hospital suffocated. Retrieved June 16, 2011 from: http://www.reuters.com/article/2011/05/24/us-usa-weather-tornadoes-hospital-idUSTRE74N.

19. Okle, S. (2008). Dr. Pou and the hurricane- implications for patient care during disasters. *New England Journal of Medicine, 358*, 1-5.

20. O'Laughlin, D. & Hick, J. (2008). Ethical issues in resource triage. *Respiratory Care, 53*, 190-200.

21. Powell ,T., Christ, K., Birkhead, G. (2008). Allocation of ventilators in a public health disaster. *Disaster Medicine and Public Health Preparedness, 2*, 20-26.

22. Simonds, A. & Sokol, D. (2009). Lives on the line? Ethics and practicalities of duty of care in pandemic and disasters. *European Respiratory Journal, 34*, 303-309.

23. Toner, E., Waldhorn, R., Maldin, B., ... O'Toole, T. (2006). Hospital preparedness for pandemic influenza. *Biosecurity and Bioterrorism: Biodefense Strategy, Practice and Science, 4*, 207-217.

# Afterword

Over the last decade, disaster response has become a subject of much discussion, both in academic and practice settings. As revealed in the literature, much of the work on disaster response and preparedness has been done since the terrorist attacks in September 2001. Many health care professionals have reported that they have had little training in this area and lack confidence and competency to effectively perform during a disaster response. There are some academic institutions offering disaster preparedness as part of their curriculum. There are other training courses through federal organizations. However, training material specifically for the profession of nursing is scant.

It is imperative that a Nurse Executive, who is responsible for nursing practice oversight, be educated about and has the tools for disaster response. As evidenced by the review of the literature, Nurse Executives need this information, but it was not readily available. It is with that lack of resource availability in mind that this toolkit was created. The intent was to include evidence from the literature, to focus on aspects for Nurse Executive competencies, and to provide a plan with resources that would enhance competent, effective, and skilled nursing practice delivery during disaster response. The toolkit includes a program plan and evaluation, training and triage models, capability assessment, and resource lists. These tools were created specifically for the Nurse Executive in an acute care setting, but could be customized for use in other areas.

Limitations may include budgetary and staffing constraints, which could hamper implementing the program plan and training. However, the defined competencies, triage model, capability assessment, and resource lists could be useful tools without full-program implementation and hands-on disaster drills.

# Appendices
# Resource Listing

# Appendix A   List of Agencies and Programs

List of

Federal Agencies, National Organizations

and

State Emergency Management Offices

# Federal Agencies & National Organizations

CDC: Center for Disease Control and Prevention—http://emergency.cdc.gov/

Department of Homeland Security—http://www.dhs.gov/files/prepresprecovery.shtm

DisasterAssistance.gov—http://www.disasterassistance.gov/daip_en.portal

FEMA: Federal Emergency Management Agency—http://www.fema.gov/

Training courses—http://www.fema.gov/emergency/nims/NIMSTrainingCourses.shtm

FDA: Food and Drug Administration—http://www.fda.gov/EmergencyPreparedness/default.htm

Medical Reserve Corps—http://www.medicalreservecorps.gov/HomePage

National Center for Medical Readiness—http://www.medicalreadiness.org/index.html

National Guard—http://www.ng.mil/default.aspx

Nuclear Regulatory Commission—http://www.nrc.gov/about-nrc/emerg-preparedness.html

Red Cross—http://www.redcross.org/

# State Agencies

Alabama Emergency Management Agency
5898 County Road 41
P.O. Drawer 2160
Clanton, Alabama 35046-2160
(205) 280-2200
(205) 280-2495 FAX
ema.alabama.gov

Alaska Division of Homeland Security and Emergency Management
P.O. Box 5750
Fort Richardson, Alaska 99505-5750
(907) 428-7000
(907) 428-7009 FAX
www.ak-prepared.com

Arizona Division of Emergency Management
5636 E. McDowell Road
Phoenix, Arizona 85008-3495
(800) 411-2336 | (602) 244-0504
(602) 464-6356 FAX
www.dem.azdema.gov

Arkansas Department of Emergency Management
Bldg. # 9501
Camp Joseph T. Robinson
North Little Rock, Arkansas 72199-9600
(501) 683-6700
(501) 683-7890 FAX
www.adem.arkansas.gov/

California Emergency Management Agency
ATTN: CSM Alex Cabassa
Training and Exercise Division
9800 Goethe Road, Box 46
Sacramento, California 95827
(916) 324-9128
(916) 324-5929 (FAX)
www.oes.ca.gov/

Colorado Division of Emergency Management
Department of Local Affairs
9195 East Mineral Avenue, Suite 200
Centennial, Colorado 80112
(720) 852-6600
(720) 852-6750 Fax
www.dola.state.co.us/ or www.coemergency.com

Connecticut Office of Emergency Management
Department of Emergency Management and Homeland Security
25 Sigourney Street 6th Floor
Hartford, Connecticut 06106-5042
(860) 256-0800
(860) 256-0815 FAX
www.ct.gov/demhs/

Delaware Emergency Management Agency
165 Brick Store Landing Road
Smyrna, Delaware 19977
(302) 659-3362
(302) 659-6855 FAX
www.dema.delaware.gov

District of Columbia Emergency Management Agency
2720 Martin Luther King, Jr. Avenue SE
Second Floor
Washington, D.C. 20032
(202) 727-6161
(202) 673-2290 FAX
dcema.dc.gov

Florida Division of Emergency Management
2555 Shumard Oak Blvd
Tallahassee, Florida 32399-2100
(850) 413-9969
(850) 488-1016 FAX
floridadisaster.org

Georgia Emergency Management Agency
935 East Confederate Avenue SE
P.O. Box 18055
Atlanta, Georgia 30316-0055
(404) 635-7000
(404) 635-7205 FAX
www.gema.state.ga.us

Hawaii State Civil Defense
3949 Diamond Head Road
Honolulu, Hawaii 96816-4495
(808) 733-4300
(808) 733-4287 FAX
www.scd.hawaii.gov

Idaho Bureau of Homeland Security
4040 Guard Street, Bldg. 600
Boise, Idaho 83705-5004
(208) 422-3040
(208) 422-3044 FAX
www.bhs.idaho.gov/

Illinois Emergency Management Agency
2200 S. Dirksen Parkway
Springfield, Illinois 62703
Office: (217) 782-2700 or (217) 782-2700
Fax: (217) 557-1978
www.state.il.us/iema

Indiana Department of Homeland Security
Indiana Government Center South
302 West Washington Street, Room E208
Indianapolis, Indiana 46204-2767
Office: (317) 232-3986
Fax: (317) 232-3895
www.in.gov/dhs

Indiana State Emergency Management Agency
302 West Washington Street
Room E-208 A
Indianapolis, Indiana 46204-2767
(317) 232-3986
(317) 232-3895 FAX
www.ai.org/sema/index.html

Iowa Homeland Security & Emergency Management Division
7105 NW 70th Avenue, Camp Dodge
Building W-4
Johnston, Iowa 50131
(515) 725-3231
(515) 281-3260 FAX
www.iowahomelandsecurity.org

Kansas Division of Emergency Management
2800 S.W. Topeka Blvd
Topeka, Kansas 66611-1287
(785) 274-1409
(785) 274-1426 FAX
www.kansas.gov/kdem

Kentucky Emergency Management
EOC Building
100 Minuteman Parkway Bldg. 100
Frankfort, Kentucky 40601-6168
(502) 607-1682 or (800) 255-2587
(502) 607-1614 FAX
www.kyem.ky.gov

Louisiana Office of Emergency Preparedness
7667 Independence Blvd
Baton Rouge, Louisiana 70806
(225) 925-7500
(225) 925-7501 FAX
www.ohsep.louisiana.gov

Maine Emergency Management Agency
#72 State House Station
45 Commerce Drive, Suite #2
Augusta, Maine 04333-0072
(207) 624-4400
(207) 287-3180 (FAX)
www.maine.gov/mema

Maryland Emergency Management Agency
Camp Fretterd Military Reservation
5401 Rue Saint Lo Drive
Reistertown, Maryland 21136
(410) 517-3600
(877) 636-2872 Toll-Free
(410) 517-3610 FAX
www.mema.state.md.us/

Massachusetts Emergency Management Agency
400 Worcester Road
Framingham, Massachusetts 01702-5399
(508) 820-2000
(508) 820-2030 FAX
www.state.ma.us/mema

Homeland Security and Emergency Management Division
Michigan Dept. of State Police
4000 Collins Road
Lansing, Michigan 48909-8136
(517) 333-5042
(517) 333-4987 FAX
www.michigan.gov/emd

Minnesota Homeland Security and Emergency Management Division
Minnesota Dept. of Public Safety
444 Cedar Street, Suite 223
St. Paul, MN 55101-6223
Office: (651) 296-0466
Fax: (651) 296-0459
www.hsem.state.mn.us

Mississippi Emergency Management Agency
P.O. Box 5644
Pearl, MS 39288-5644
(601) 933-6362
(800) 442-6362 Toll Free
(601) 933-6800 FAX
www.msema.org

Missouri Emergency Management Agency
2302 Militia Drive
P.O. Box 116
Jefferson City, Missouri 65102
(573) 526-9100
(573) 634-7966 FAX
sema.dps.mo.gov
JFHQ-MT

Montana Division of Disaster & Emergency Services
1956 Mt Majo Street
PO BOX 4789
Fort Harrison, Montana 59636-4789
(406) 841-3911
(406) 841-3965 FAX
www.dma.mt.gov/des/

Nebraska Emergency Management Agency
1300 Military Road
Lincoln, Nebraska 68508-1090
(402) 471-7421
(402) 471-7433 FAX
www.nema.ne.gov

Nevada Division of Emergency Management
2478 Fairview Drive
Carson City, Nevada 89701
(775) 687-0300
(775) 687-0330 FAX
www.dem.state.nv.us/

Governor's Office of Emergency Management
State Office Park South
33 Hazen Drive
Concord, New Hampshire 03305
(603) 271-2231
(603) 271-3609 FAX
www.nh.gov/safety/divisions/bem

New Jersey Office of Emergency Management
Emergency Management Bureau
P.O. Box 7068
West Trenton, New Jersey 08628-0068
(609) 538-6050 Monday-Friday
(609) 584-5000
(609) 584-1528 FAX
www.ready.nj.gov

## Appendices Resource Listing

New Mexico Department of Homeland Security
and Emergency Management (DHSEM)
13 Bataan Blvd
P.O. Box 27111
Santa Fe, New Mexico 87502
(505) 476-9600
(505) 476-9635 Emergency
(505) 476-9695 FAX
www.nmdhsem.org/

New York State Emergency Management Office
1220 Washington Avenue
Building 22, Suite 101
Albany, New York 12226-2251
(518) 292-2275
(518) 322-4978 FAX
www.semo.state.ny.us/

North Carolina Division of Emergency Management
4713 Mail Service Center
Raleigh, NC 27699-4713
(919) 733-3867
(919) 733-5406 FAX
www.ncem.org/

North Dakota Department of Emergency Services
P.O. Box 5511
Bismarck, North Dakota 58506-5511
(701) 328-8100
(701) 328-8181 FAX
www.nd.gov/des

Ohio Emergency Management Agency
2855 West Dublin-Granville Road
Columbus, Ohio 43235-2206
Office: (614) 889-7150
Fax: (614) 889-7183
ww.ema.ohio.gov/ema.asp

Oklahoma Department of Emergency Management
2401 Lincoln Blvd Suite C51
Oklahoma City, Oklahoma 73105
(405) 521-2481
(405) 521-4053 FAX
http://www.ok.gov/OEM/

Oregon Emergency Management
Department of State Police
3225 State Street
Salem, Oregon 97309-5062
(503) 378-2911
(503) 373-7833 FAX
www.oregon.gov/OMD/OEM/index.shtml

Pennsylvania Emergency Management Agency
2605 Interstate Drive
Harrisburg PA 17110-9463
(717) 651-2001
(717) 651-2040 FAX
www.pema.state.pa.us/

Rhode Island Emergency Management Agency
645 New London Avenue
Cranston, Rhode Island 02920-3003
(401) 946-9996
(401) 944-1891 FAX
www.riema.ri.gov

South Carolina Emergency Management Division
2779 Fish Hatchery Road
West Columbia South Carolina 29172
(803) 737-8500
(803) 737-8570 FAX
www.scemd.org/

South Dakota Division of Emergency Management
118 West Capitol
Pierre, South Dakota 57501
(605) 773-3231
(605) 773-3580 FAX
www.oem.sd.gov

Tennessee Emergency Management Agency
3041 Sidco Drive
Nashville, Tennessee 37204-1502
(615) 741-0001
(615) 242-9635 FAX
www.tnema.org

Texas Division of Emergency Management
5805 N. Lamar Blvd
PO BOX 4087
Austin, Texas 78773-0220
(512) 424-2138
(512) 424-2444 or 7160 FAX www.txdps.state.tx.us/dem/

Utah Division of Emergency Services and Homeland Security
1110 State Office Building
P.O. Box 141710
Salt Lake City, Utah 84114-1710
(801) 538-3400
(801) 538-3770 FAX
www.des.utah.gov

Vermont Emergency Management Agency
Department of Public Safety
Waterbury State Complex
103 South Main Street
Waterbury, Vermont 05671-2101
(802) 244-8721
(800) 347-0488
(802) 244-8655 FAX
www.dps.state.vt.us/vem/

Virginia Department of Emergency Management
10501 Trade Court
Richmond, VA 23236-3713
(804) 897-6500
(804) 897-6556 FAX
www.vaemergency.com

State of Washington Emergency Management Division
Building 20, M/S: TA-20
Camp Murray, Washington 98430-5122
(253) 512-7000
(800) 562-6108
(253) 512-7200 FAX
www.emd.wa.gov/

West Virginia Office of Emergency Services
Building 1, Room EB-80 1900 Kanawha Blvd, East
Charleston, West Virginia 25305-0360
(304) 558-5380
(304) 344-4538 FAX
www.wvdhsem.gov

Wisconsin Emergency Management
2400 Wright Street
P.O. Box 7865
Madison, Wisconsin 53707-7865
Phone: (608) 242-3232
Fax: (608) 242-3247
emergencymanagement.wi.gov/

Wyoming Office of Homeland Security
Herschler Bldg. 1st Floor East
122 W. 25th Street
Cheyenne, Wyoming 82002
(307) 777-4663
(307) 635-6017 FAX
wyohomelandsecurity.state.wy.us

# Appendix B
# Academic Programs

# Academic Programs That Offer Training Courses and Degrees

Albert Einstein Healthcare Network—http://www.einstein.edu/education/programs/25-cur/ems-&-disaster-medicine.html

American Military University—http://www.amu.apus.edu/lp/emergency-and-disaster-management/

Columbia University—http://www.ncdp.mailman.columbia.edu/training.htm

Empire State College—http://www8.esc.edu/esconline/across_esc/cdl/cdl.nsf/home.html

George Washington University—http://www.gwu.edu/~icdrm/index.html

Johns Hopkins—http://www.jhsph.edu/refugee/education_training/degrees/

Johns Hopkins Nursing—http://www.ijhn.jhmi.edu/contEd_3rdLevel_Class.asp?id=EmerPrepareHome&numContEdID=6

Louisiana State University—http://sdmi.lsu.edu/disaster_response.html

Missouri State University—http://www.missouristate.edu/human/training/safety.htm

National Domestic Preparedness Consortium (NDPC)—http://www.ndpc.us/index.html

New Mexico Tech—http://www.emrtc.nmt.edu/training/

Philadelphia University—http://www.philau.edu/disastermed/index.htm

Rural Domestic Preparedness Consortium—http://www.ruraltraining.org/about

Rutgers University—http://rues.rutgers.edu/cert.shtml

Stanford University—CoOL Disaster Preparedness and Response

http://cool.conservation-us.org/bytopic/disasters/

Texas Department of State Health Services—http://www.dshs.state.tx.us/comprep/training/Online-Training-Opportunities-and-Resources/

University of Copenhagen—http://www.mdma.ku.dk/

University of Findlay—http://emergency-management-training.findlay.edu/

University of Hawaii—http://ndptc.hawaii.edu/

University of Maryland Baltimore County—http://ehs.umbc.edu/CEEDR1

University of North Carolina Center for Public Health Preparedness—http://cphp.sph.unc.edu/training/nc_drn/

University of Oregon—http://emc.uoregon.edu/content/training

University of Peshawar Pakistan—http://www.auedm.net/Data/activities/1st%20Workshop/Workshop/Aslam%20Khan/Master%20of%20Disaster%20presentation%20July%202008%20final.pdf

University of Pittsburgh—http://www.prepare.pitt.edu/

University of South Florida, Center for Public Health Preparedness—http://www.fcphp.usf.edu/courselistings/courses_ListingsBFAST.htm

University of South Florida, College of Nursing—http://hsc.usf.edu/nocms/nursing/docs/research/BTTrainingProgram.pdf

University of Utah—http://www.health.utah.edu/healthpromotion/cep/Disaster%20Response.html

University of Wisconsin-Madison—http://dmc.engr.wisc.edu/

Vanderbilt University—http://www.nursing.vanderbilt.edu/incmce/overview.html

Western Carolina University—http://www.wcu.edu/5719.asp

Yale New Haven Health—http://ynhhs.emergencyeducation.org/

www.ingramcontent.com/pod-product-compliance
Lightning Source LLC
Chambersburg PA
CBHW041059180526
45172CB00001B/23